Penny Clarke is a qualified step instructor, having attended classes since the fitness programme first took off in the UK. She read English at Nottingham University, obtaining a First, and is now an editor in a Scottish publishing company. She is scorer for the Reivers baseball team, a club she helped set up in 1989.

the ultimate step

Penny Clarke

Foreword by Connie Williams,
Originator of Bench Stepping

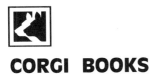

CORGI BOOKS

A CORGI BOOK 0 552 13970 X

First publication in Great Britain

PRINTING HISTORY
Corgi edition published 1993

This book is set in 11 on 13 Garamond 3

Corgi Books are published by Transworld Publishers Ltd, 61-63
Uxbridge Road, Ealing, London W5 5SA, in Australia by Transworld
Publishers (Australia) Pty Ltd, 15-23 Helles Avenue, Moorebank, NS
2170, and in New Zealand by Transworld Publishers (NZ) Ltd, 3 Will
Pickering Drive, Albany, Auckland.

Made and printed in Great Britain by
William Clowes Limited, Beccles, Suffolk.

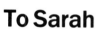

To Sarah

contents

acknowledgements

I would like to thank the following people for helping me to write this book: my editors, Averil Ashfield and Judy Moir, for their care and attention in working on the manuscript; Guy Feldman of Area 5 Productions, Edinburgh, for the (over-extended) use of his PC and printer — thanks; John Philip, for his patience in teaching me how to use it, and his good humour when taking the hundred-odd photos for Irene Barry's excellent illustrations; Ryan Orr, for posing so well; Sue Maic, for her support and great suggestions in the nutrition chapter; Donald Eunson, for his unique disk drive; Connie Williams of Bench-aerobix, for all her support and encouragement from her base in Atlanta, Georgia; and Jim Coleman and Lynne Denham, Step Reebok instructors extraordinaire, for unwittingly inspiring me to write all this in the first place. And finally, I'd like to say a big thank-you to my family, especially Dad and my sister Sarah. And of course, a big thank-you to Donald.

foreword

By Connie Williams

Originator of Bench Stepping

U P, UP, DOWN, down . . . up, up, down, down . . . up, up, down, down . . . It sounds like a military march, but no . . . it's bench aerobics.

Who would have thought that something as elementary as stepping up and down could have revolutionized the fitness industry? Until five years ago, certainly not me.

In January 1987 I resigned from my position in sales, marketing and product development with a large Japanese children's company. I had held this job for four years — four years of travelling and keeping up an unbelievable schedule which involved entertaining clients, eating out — or not eating at all — and certainly having no time to exercise. All of which led to a 20lb weight gain. I was miserable. I was raised an athlete — played every sport, danced tap and ballet, gymnastics — you name it, I did it. I was never still for one minute and, of course, was never overweight. However, I

was now no longer in my element, so I left my company and decided to go back to school to study exercise physiology and do something with my jelly legs.

I went back to teaching aerobics, started a weight-training programme and began to work with clients one to one to design personal fitness programmes. I saw great results from my weight-training programme, but the aerobics classes were killing my body. My knees hurt, my shins hurt, my ankles hurt, my back hurt. After a year, I was considering giving up aerobics altogether.

Suddenly a stair-climbing machine appeared in our club, and it immediately became the most sought-after piece of equipment there. Everyone wanted to climb on it . . . even me with all my aches and pains. In fact, the stair-climber became so popular that a sign-up sheet was introduced and people were limited to 20-minute sessions.

It occurred to me that the reason for the

success of this machine and this form of exercise was that everyone was just like me. They knew the importance of aerobic exercise, but high-impact forms were killing them and the low-impact was just not intense enough.

Voilà! The stair-climbing machine. It is low-impact and, operated correctly, provides a very intense cardiovascular workout. It also uses body-weight resistance, which will give you muscle tone and strength in your lower body – and let's face it, most people want to burn fat and tone up this area. The only problem was that we didn't have enough machines to go round.

I began to invite my aerobics students to the instructor's stage, to step up and down for about five minutes of each class. The students liked it so much that we began to increase our time here, varying our stepping patterns.

Soon I was able to persuade the owner of the club to build me more stages to accommodate the growing number of students interested in stage-climbing. Ten stages were built at a cost of about $100 (£50) each. The dimensions were 8 feet long by 3 feet wide and they ranged in height from 12 inches to 16 inches. They were carpeted and weighed about 50–60 lb, and each could accommodate three people, so we had room enough for 30 students. They looked like benches and from this came the name – 'BenchAerobix'.

A total of 48 students signed up for my first class, which was the largest class attendance in over a year. SUCCESS! We had a programme that worked. The owners of the club scurried around building more benches, while I scurried around training more instructors to teach this new form of workout. Almost overnight bench-stepping aerobics classes took over the entire schedule, because that was what everyone wanted. What we had done was take the concept of the stair-climbing machine into an aerobics-room environment.

It was not a new idea. Athletes have been climbing stadium stairs for years. It just came at a time when people were leaving aerobics classes in search of alternative exercise programmes. They had become bored and/or injured and were not getting the changes they were hoping for in their bodies – just maintaining them the way they were. BenchAerobix helped to push them into a higher, more challenging mode of fitness training, and everyone was ready for the change and the push – or should I say climb – to get there.

I attribute the success of this programme to the fact that BenchAerobix gave its students RESULTS. People started changing their bodies as never before in any other form of exercise they had tried – changes they could see and feel. Friends, family, colleagues: everyone who saw them noticed the difference. Now the hour they had been spending every day exercising was paying off. Their hips, thighs and buttocks were tighter, smaller and more toned. Yes, results . . . that was what they wanted, that was what they got. That is success.

As for me, I was bombarded with phone calls from all over the country to teach clubs and instructors how to implement the programme. I designed a smaller version of the bench to accommodate the individual stepper in order to get more people into a class, and I soon became business partners with a friend and formed a company called Bench Blast Inc. We taught anyone who would listen to us. And to be quite honest, we were astonished by the acceptance of the fitness industry and the programme's unbelievable success. To think that a little idea could blossom and revolutionize an industry and change so many people's lives is almost incredible and has been truly overwhelming.

My original business partner in Bench Blast Inc. eventually took a position with a well-known shoe company to head their step-training programme. I decided to keep my own company intact and chose another business partner to form BenchAerobix Inc. We market our video and bench products worldwide and I continue to train instructors on the proper techniques of the programme.

Sometimes I think I was crazy or that this has all been a dream — even a nightmare at times. But I am grateful to have been part of this adventure on life's journey — and thankful for the opportunities of sharing my love for and knowledge of this programme with the world.

I hope that this book will prove an inspiration for you, helping you to have the body you have always wanted. I know that this programme works and I know it will work for you.

Always remember — every step you take to train your body, mind and spirit brings you closer to your dreams.

Enjoy!

Connie Williams
Atlanta, Georgia

chapter one

Introducing Benchwork

The Habit of a Lifetime

TAKE ONE LOW bench, some good music and a desire to do something about your overall level of fitness, and you've got all the ingredients for a challenging and effective workout. Or at least, that was my first impression having wandered past Studio One at my local leisure centre one day and seen the somewhat surreal vision of about 30 or 40 sweaty people on individual benches, marching up and down in time to the music while a woman at the front yelled, 'Tap down!' The woman was Lynne Denham, the programme was bench stepping, and I've been hooked ever since.

And that surprised me too. I've always been sceptical about the business of fitness, and I've never *really* enjoyed a conventional aerobics class. Sure, my heart pounded and my muscles ached, but for all that effort and heavy breathing I never seemed to change shape. And I'm not the type to do something for the sake of it without visible proof that it's doing me some good.

So, if you're the type of person whose lungs instinctively heave at the very mention of 'aerobics', or the thought of dancing around a crowded room leaves you absolutely cold, take heart. Step training is simple and adaptable. And it gets results.

At its most basic level, benchwork involves no more than stepping on and off a low platform. Simple. But the very action of lifting your body upward and forward against the force of gravity uses the major muscles in the lower body to create a big demand on the most important muscle of all – your heart. And when you train and strengthen this muscle, you reduce the amount of work it has to do to perform effectively. More than that, stepping also strengthens and conditions those lower-body muscles at the same time, visibly toning up the hips, buttocks and thighs. Then add some simple arm exercises to tone and strengthen your upper body, and you've got a safe programme which caters for cardiorespiratory endurance, strength, co-ordination, balance and agility — and all in one time-efficient package. Of course, it would be great if everybody had hours to spend down at the gym or at a barrage of different fitness classes, but we don't. A couple of hours a week is often the most that we can manage. So if one session on a bench uses and improves a far greater range of fitness elements than other forms of exercise, we'll do it.

Benchwork is a 'low-impact' form of exercise, fitness-speak for a programme in which one foot is always on the floor so that the risk of stress-related injury through jarring on the muscles and joints is reduced to a minimum. Indeed, studies carried out at San Diego State University have shown that the stress on the body during step training is equivalent to walking at 3 mph — while the oxygen or calorific cost is similar to jogging at as much as 7 mph. Impressive stuff. Benchwork may well be soft on the joints but it's no soft option, and it's only the amount that you sweat which gives you any real indication of how hard you're actually working. For once the music starts and you're well warmed up, you're off — marching through a non-stop series of simple step patterns and exercises, which maintain your heart rate at a steady level but never become uncomfortable. So smokers beware! You've got no excuse now, because a well-orchestrated workout should not overtax your lungs.

Why *The Ultimate Step*? For the simple reason that it's sometimes very difficult to find out any information about step training — why certain techniques are advocated, what differences the use of handweights actually make, if it is really as safe and effective a form of exercise as all the hype suggests. Part of the problem here is that objective research into benchwork is yet in its infancy and, although bench-stepping has been around for some years in one form or another, as a specific programme set to music it is still very new. So with this in mind, the following chapters aim to set out the type of information that should help you understand not only *what* a benchwork programme is all about in terms of the type of foot- and armwork involved, but *why* it works as an effective form of fitness training and *how* you can enhance your performance by approaching it sensibly and making a few minor adjustments to your lifestyle. Yes, *The Ultimate Step* also includes a few words about eating for energy — although it's very definitely *not* a diet chapter. Self-denial is not my thing. However, you may well find that a few simple adjustments to your food make all the difference between a half-hearted workout and one which gets maximum results.

Benchwork is as challenging as you choose to make it. Indeed, it's refreshing to see so many men taking part; this type of programme has laid to rest the myth that aerobics is a female domain and in some way an easy option. For whether you're the most firmly rooted couch potato or a performance athlete in training, you can get as much or as little from the routine as you want. And be it in the privacy of your own living-room or as part of a class, *The Ultimate Step* will help you improve your level of cardiorespiratory fitness, burn fat, tone and strengthen you up — and leave you coming back for more.

How to Use
The Ultimate Step

Before launching yourself wholeheartedly into the steps and routines, it's important to read through Chapters Two to Four containing an assortment of facts and useful information. You'll quickly get used to the jargon of benchwork – the world of tap downs and straddle/squats, traverses and side legs – and if you have already been to a step class or two, you may well know some of these exercises and movements by different names. Nevertheless, to end all confusion and make the book as easy to follow as possible, there is a Glossary on p112 covering the most common terms.

In every chapter which involves actual stepping, the various exercises are described in full at the start so that you can practise the moves and perfect your technique. A routine then follows using the step patterns you've just learned, and these are then summarized in Appendix 2 so that you can follow them more easily.

Then comes a cool-down section, to bring your pulse rate down to a more normal level and stretch your body out after all that exertion. This is followed by a simple chapter on strength training which is suitable for beginners and seasoned steppers alike. You can *either* do the strength training at the end of your workout – in which case you should simply wind your body down a bit and save your stretches for the very end – or you can do these exercises independently if you fancy toning yourself up but don't feel like a full-blown step routine one day. The choice is yours, and *The Ultimate Step* is designed to be as flexible as possible.

chapter two

A Workout for Everyone

Adapting the Routine to Meet Your Needs

THE CLAIMS MADE about benchwork make good reading. Short of putting the cat out and turning lead into gold, it sometimes seems that there's nothing step can't do – and that includes prolonging your life expectancy. Of course, step training, like any aerobic exercise, *can* help prolong your life expectancy: it will maintain your body – your heart, lungs, muscles and bones – in a good state of health, and can play an active role in the prevention and control of many diseases and debilitating illnesses such as coronary heart disease and osteoporosis (brittle bone disease). Not only that, but as with all forms of aerobic exercise, chemicals called endorphins are released into your brain when you step, producing a sense of well-being – I can certainly vouch for benchwork being an excellent form of stress relief. And take my word for it for now, maybe, but energy produces energy. Start working out regularly and you'll have a lot more bounce and enthusiasm in everything you do.

But that's the longer-term view. It's what's happening in the short term that most people want to know about – the here and now and maybe tomorrow if you really have to wait that long. That's what counts when you're running for the bus and, more important still for many people, that's what matters when you're basking on a beach or pouring yourself into your once-favourite trousers. In other words, the thing most people want to know about a new exercise programme is how quickly they will get results.

The Burning Question

Since the earliest days, when Connie Williams's first-ever classes were oversubscribed and you had to make do with a slot on the stair-climbing machine, benchwork's success as a form of aerobic exercise has proved irresistible – not least because of its obvious potential as a method of altering the balance between fat and muscle on the body. People wanted to know more. Researchers became fascinated by this new fitness phenomenon; manufacturers wanted the statistics to bolster their advertising campaigns. So it is not, perhaps, surprising that, having started their comprehensive bench-stepping programme, shoe manufacturers Reebok were among the first to commission formal research into the biomechanics of step training, paving the way for many further and varied studies.

A Question of Calories

There are clearly a lot of variables to consider when estimating the energy cost of a benchwork routine. At the most basic level, physical factors like the bench-height you use, your body weight and the choreography employed all affect the amount of energy a given workout will use. Similarly, some people seek benchwork's ability to give their cardiorespiratory system a run for its money while others exploit its cross-training potential by incorporating it into interval training – three minutes stepping, three minutes strength work and so on. A magic number for calories burnt no more exists than an 'average' step routine, but at least knowing the variables can help you to adapt the intensity of your workout to suit your individual needs.

Bench-height

The height of your platform drastically affects the intensity of your routine. Obviously, the higher you step, the harder it is, and raising your bench just two inches can increase the energy cost of your workout by anything from under 1 calorie a minute to over 2, depending on your weight. The heavier you are, the more energy it takes to do a given routine. Now, talking in terms of burning an extra 1–2 calories

a minute might not sound all that much, but it's equivalent to about 20–60 calories over a half-hour workout and believe me, it'll feel a lot harder almost immediately.

Steps per Minute

It also makes sense that the more times you step up and down every minute, the more energy you use up, and again, the smallest increase in tempo from one record to the next can make your workout seem that much harder. However, benchwork is not intended to be a race, and while some instructors will pitch their classes at as many as 130 beats per minute, a slower pace of between 118–124 bpm is more than sufficient and is also the approximate step rate on which the table on p6 is based.

Choreography

Similarly, the type of step patterns you use can drastically affect your workrate. The static straight step with a leading leg (up-up-down-down), on which all beginner's routines are based, seems exhausting when you first start. But it really doesn't take long for your body to demand a more intense workout, and when the more vigorous lunges, travelling steps and repeaters are introduced, working the bench from all angles and attacking virtually every muscle in your lower body, you'll look back to those first routines with a certain degree of fondness – and gloat that you can now do them and hardly break sweat!

Armed and Ready

On top of that comes the armwork, and from recent research carried out by Goss et al. at the University of Pittsburgh it can be estimated that a given workout involving vigorous arm movements is as much as 15 per cent more demanding than that same routine executed without any arm movements – especially if the exercises include a lot of strong vertical motions like shoulder presses (see p49). Similarly, step's much-celebrated adaptability for use with small handweights again contributes to an increased demand on your body.

The Energy Cost of Stepping

I have drawn up a table to illustrate the number of calories (energy cost) burned in a 30-minute step routine which is executed at 120 bpm. The table is based on figures reported by Tony Lycholat in *Asset*, January 1992, for the calorific demand of the Step Reebok programme.

The lower figure in each entry refers to the energy consumption of a basic workout, using the most simple of steps without any arm movements, while the upper figure refers to a vigorous workout which makes full use of the bench and the most demanding foot and

arm movements. Given the number of variables already cited, though, these calculations provide no more than an *approximate* guide to the type of levels involved and should not be taken as gospel. They are, nevertheless, impressive and you can see immediately why benchwork is such a challenging form of aerobic exercise.

If these calculations *still* don't convince you, according to the 1991 American College of Sports Medicine (ACSM) *Guidelines for Exercise Testing and Prescription*, step exercise is equivalent to:

● jogging at 5–7 mph
● cycling at 10–15 mph (without a head wind)

in terms of calorific or oxygen cost per minute. I know which I find most interesting. Similarly, when it comes to changing your body's composition – the ratio of fat to muscle – benchwork fares well. Preliminary studies seem to show that step training does decrease the body fat percentage significantly – I, and thousands of others, will vouch for that any day – and anyone who knows a step fanatic can't fail to have seen the dramatic effect this type of workout has on

The Energy Cost of Stepping

| step height | | workrate | calories (kcal) burned in 30 minutes for various body weights | | | | | | |
imp.	metric	METs*	7 stone 44.4 kg	8 stone 50.8 kg	9 stone 57.1 kg	10 stone 63.5 kg	11 stone 69.8 kg	12 stone 76.2 kg	13 stone 82.5 kg
4"	10 cm	5–7.5	110–170	130–190	140–210	160–240	170–260	190–290	210–310
6"	15 cm	6–9	130–200	150–230	170–260	190–290	210–310	230–340	250–370
8"	20 cm	7–10.5	150–230	180–270	200–300	220–330	240–360	270–400	290–430

*This is the rate of energy use, MET being the abbreviation of Metabolic Equivalent and 1 MET representing the approximate amount of oxygen consumed in a minute by someone just sitting quietly. In other words, if you do a

vigorous 30-minute step routine on a 6-inch bench, you will consume up to nine times the amount of oxygen – and hence nine times the energy – that you would if you spent that same half-hour staring at the TV.

trimming down and toning up the hips, buttocks and thighs while conditioning and strengthening the upper body. The oft-quoted statistic of step training reducing body fat by 30 per cent more than other forms of dance-orientated aerobics should be taken with a pinch of salt, though, since everybody's metabolism is different, and while this result was achieved under strict laboratory conditions when research into benchwork first began, it is now generally agreed to be a somewhat optimistic figure.

So, secure in the knowledge that bench-stepping will help condition your cardiorespiratory system, reduce those fat deposits and tone and strengthen you up, it's time to look a little more closely at how you go about it.

Use Your Head

As with all fitness programmes, you must be sensible when approaching a bench-stepping workout, and if, for example, you are very overweight, have problems with your knees or ankles, are pregnant, smoke heavily or have some sort of heart or respiratory condition – in other words, if you *know* that you should take things a bit easy – you should obviously seek medical advice before proceeding any further.

Most people can begin stepping straight away, though, and, as long as you listen to your body and always watch out for telltale signs of overexertion, you should have no problem with the programme. As Brassey and partners point out, 'Exercise becomes a hazard when warning symptoms are ignored, participation is erratic or the intensity or duration reaches a level which involves distress rather than discomfort' (*Practitioner*, December 1987, Volume 231). If you do experience difficulty in breathing, have an irregular heartbeat, chest pain, dizziness or even a sudden lack of co-ordination or nausea,

common sense will tell you to visit your doctor straight away. And if by chance you do happen to injure yourself while stepping, don't be a martyr and battle on regardless. You'll only make the problem worse and end up having to take a far longer break from exercise than originally necessary – which won't help your level of fitness one bit.

How Long and How Often?

Warning – benchwork can be addictive! Try it once and nine times out of ten you're hooked. There's no rhyme nor reason to this – after all, it's a pretty strange way to spend your time and, considering how hard it makes you work, it is, perhaps, remarkable that people come, and keep on coming back, time after time.

On the other hand, if you must become addicted to something, there are definitely worse habits to pick up than one which develops your level of fitness in the way benchwork does. Nevertheless, the warning still holds. It's all too easy to become obsessed – stepping day in and day out, increasing the intensity little by little, seeking that feeling of satisfied exhilaration but never really giving your body sufficient time to recover. Rest is as important a part of training as activity. Your body needs at least a couple of days off a week to rebuild your depleted energy levels and consolidate your progress so far, and this is one of the reasons the ACSM (*Guidelines*) recommend that a maximum of five days' exercise of this nature a week are more than sufficient to improve your cardiorespiratory fitness.

For me, though, three testing workouts a week are enough. Four, and I immediately feel that I'm not putting as much into them as I could, compromising on my technique and becoming lazy about controlling and really working my arms. Anyway, if you're anything like me, rationing yourself in this way will make you look forward to your step-training sessions all the more.

Similarly, when it comes to the length of time spent actually stepping in your workouts, take things gradually. The ACSM (*Guidelines*) advise that to benefit from aerobic training you should work towards the upper limit of your individual capacity (see below) for between 15 and 60 minutes, *depending on how hard you are working* – a useful qualifying statement to make. Benchwork demands a lot from your body. If it's your first time, 15 minutes' step training will be more than enough to be going on with. So warm up, do your quarter of an hour and then cool down again. And only when you have mastered the technique and introduced your body to the new demands that you are making of it, begin building up the amount of time spent actually stepping to 20, then 25, then 30 minutes and so on. Believe me, put everything into that quarter- or half-hour session and you'll get more than a thorough workout!

How High and How Quickly?

Whether using a manufactured bench or adapting a box or crate for the purpose (see Chapter Three), the most significant way of altering the intensity of your workout is by raising or lowering the height of your step. Manufactured benches range in two-inch intervals from four inches (10cm) in height to a potential maximum of twelve (30cm), and, I must admit, when I first started out it really did seem as if there was some kind of competition to see who could step with the highest bench for the longest amount of time and still live to tell the tale. However, the object of the step training is not to play some masochistic form of higher and higher but to find the bench-height at which you personally work

most effectively. And irrespective of how tall you are, there is no real reason to work on anything higher than eight inches.

That being said, though, knowing at what height to start stepping and then how fast to progress from level to level can be difficult. If this is the first time you've emerged from your armchair in many years, there's nothing to stop you practising the footwork and arm movements for a few sessions without using a bench at all – an ideal breaking-in period, enjoying the privacy of your own living room. Indeed, if you do then decide to try out the local leisure centre, at least you'll know what you're letting yourself in for and will find your first class session far less intimidating. However, even if you consider yourself relatively fit, start on no more than a four- or six-inch step and don't be in a hurry to raise it.

According to ACSM, you'll notice the most significant effects of your fitness conditioning within six to eight weeks of beginning training. Brassey and partners advise that all exercise programmes should increase in intensity in small stages – each stage taking eight to ten weeks, particularly if you are elderly or very unfit. An increase of two inches might not sound that much but believe me, it can feel mountainous, and only when you are absolutely confident at a given height – working your arms vigorously and attacking your routine right to the very end – should you even consider taking on the next step. Besides, you can always lower your bench again after about fifteen minutes if you find it too demanding, so enjoy this transitionary period – and when you do finally manage the whole routine on your new height, you'll feel great. Remember – there's nothing to stop you going back to your old height if you're feeling tired during one workout, or maybe fancy focusing on your upper body a bit more fully instead of simply your legs. All you've done is open up a few more options.

Increasing the bench-height to ten, even twelve inches will obviously make your workout all the more challenging, and I freely admit that there is something very appealing about the total sweat approach. However, it may well have a detrimental effect on other areas in your routine – compromising your posture, for instance, which will in turn throw everything else out – so you could well find that your desire to push yourself to the limit is increasing your risk of injury dramatically. Remember – you can always increase the length of time spent stepping if you want to raise the demand of your workout more safely.

Intensity – The Heart of Training

Measuring how hard you are working is probably the most important factor of all to check. You may be working out several times a week and monitoring how long each session lasts but, especially if you are exercising at home where there is no instructor keeping an eye on you, the *intensity* of your routine is more difficult to gauge. Too easy, and you won't achieve the full benefits that cardiorespiratory fitness can bring; too hard, and you become painfully short of breath, feel a pounding in your chest, increase the risk of injury since your technique will tend to suffer, and become exhausted, sore and stiff – any one of which is enough to put you off exercising for life!

Your Target Heart Rate

The most accurate way for you to assess the intensity of your workout is to measure your heart rate. Obviously, the more times it beats

per minute, the harder you are exercising because your body's requiring more energy. But before you actually start step training it is important to calculate your own individual 'training' or 'target heart rate' – THR (see Appendix 1) – and then keep an eye on your pulse during your routine. If it's on the low side according to your calculation, increase the intensity with a few, more vigorous foot patterns like lunges and repeaters (see p50), or maybe work your upper body harder with arm movements like lateral raises or flyes (see pp39–40); on the high side you should lower the height of your bench if you can, or alternatively place your hands on your hips for a while or even return to the simple up-up-down-down step with your hands swinging loosely by your sides until your pulse has slowed down a bit. You should be aiming at a level of intensity which feels somewhere between a 'moderate' demand on your body and a 'heavy' demand (see Appendix 1) – so if your heart is thundering and your lungs fit to burst, you're overdoing it a bit!

A Question of Muscle

Benchwork's ability to tone and build muscle has been an advertiser's dream. Step training has taken off at precisely the time when the well-defined physique is in great demand, and bench manufacturers have not been slow to cash in on this lucrative angle, employing punchy slogans stressing strength and power with the help of well-toned models bearing handweights and sweat. However, before you rush straight off and start pumping away with the weights for all you're worth, pause a moment for thought. For there is strength training and there is strength training, and simply adding weight to your normal routine may not be the best way of achieving better muscle definition and strength.

Studies do indicate that you can increase the energy expenditure of a given step routine by 1–3 calories per minute by adding two-pound handweights. In practice, though, two pounds is a lot of weight to be shifting around for a full vigorous workout – I certainly couldn't do it – and unless you are an extremely experienced and physically strong stepper, the chances are that your technique will suffer as you try to compensate for the extra effort involved. Thus, you are increasing the risk of injury dramatically, and the moment you have to slow the pace of your routine to accommodate the added weight, the energy cost will drop.

However, using small handweights, conditioning bands or one of the new strength-training devices like the Step Strap or V-Toner as part of a specific muscle-toning programme using your bench is a different matter, and Chapter Ten provides an introduction to the way strength training can be added on to the end of your workout, without risking your technique or compromising the aerobic demand of your actual step routines. So, for the purposes of this book, keep the handweights locked away until that point, and just concentrate on the correct and vigorous execution of the steps and arm movements outlined from Chapter Four onwards.

Myth, Magic or Sheer Hard Work?

When all is said and done, there is nothing magical about benchwork, and if you're looking for an instant cure for that comforting bulge about your waistline, think twice. Step training does substantially reduce body fat, is an excellent method of strengthening and toning yourself up – especially around the dreaded hips, buttocks and thighs – and it will improve the efficiency of your heart considerably. But it's sheer hard work that makes this happen; the magic is that the very process of stepping, combined with good strong music, seems in some way to distract you from realizing how hard you are actually working. And just in case you're interested, if you do just the simple up-up-down-down step on an eight-inch bench for half an hour at 120 beats per minute, you will actually be climbing up and down 600 feet – the equivalent of marching halfway up the Empire State Building and back. Put it like that, and it's a miracle anyone even thinks about step training!

chapter three

Tools of the Trade

Equipment — Essential and Otherwise

THERE IS NOTHING worse than trying some form of exercise for the first time and not feeling the part. It's bad enough that you don't really know what's going on and strongly suspect that you have two left feet, without having to worry about the finer points of dress. Two distinct groups of people seem to appear — those who rush out and buy themselves the hottest new range of aerobics gear before they start, and those who make do and mend like I did, raking their cupboards for something vaguely appropriate while being acutely aware that canvas baseball boots aren't really quite the right thing to wear and that you probably will be rather hot in heavy-duty sweat pants.

Nevertheless, spending a fortune on gear is no guarantee that you'll feel any less conspicuous during your first workout. Indeed, the reason most people take up aerobic exercise is to try and lose a bit of excess body fat, and coating yourself in a clingy layer of Lycra which leaves no bump

unexposed is hardly flattering. So while wearing appropriate clothes is important, especially when it comes to footwear, don't rush out and buy anything until you are sure that you're going to continue. There are plenty of ways of spending the money when you really do become hooked later on!

Top to Toe

Of course, if you subscribe to the school of thought of Suzan Stadner in her *Intimate Workout for Lovers*, you don't even have to think about boring old leotards and restricting bike shorts, but can throw caution to the wind and work out stark naked. However, you'll definitely get the net curtains twitching if you're exercising at home, and you may well find more than the odd eyebrow raised if you try it at your local leisure centre. Despite the fact that step is a low-impact form of exercise, it's still a vigorous workout and not everyone has gravity-resistant breasts and swing-proof genitalia.

So if this extreme of aerobic freedom is not to your taste, add layers accordingly. And as long as you're cool and comfortable, it doesn't matter what you wear. Remember –

- **loose-fitting T-shirts hide a multitude of sins, can double up as a convenient way to mop your sweaty brow, and stop you sliding off your bench during the abdominal work**
- **some form of chest support is definitely worth thinking about for women – irrespective of size, believe me!**
- **G-string bottoms creep upward in direct proportion to the height of your bench**
- **jock straps are a must for men – whether baggy sweats or leave-nothing-to-the-imagination bike shorts are your thing**
- **and good absorbent socks can help prevent your trainers from becoming too unsavoury.**

The Sole of Stepping

One thing that's definitely worth investing in is a good pair of training shoes – you simply cannot pad around in bare feet during benchwork. Support and cushioning are essential and, if the shoes are the right ones for the job, you really will notice the difference they make to your workout, not to mention helping to prevent injury to the lower leg.

There are now several custom-designed step-training shoes available on the market. All are extremely light (between 7–9 oz each, or 200–250 g), have low heel collars (the bit running round behind your ankle) and are often made from breathable, washable material. Consumer-friendly to the last.

However, the drawback with aerobics shoes is that the soles are designed for indoor surfaces and won't last very long if used for jogging or any other form of outside sport. You might be better off with a 'cross trainer' instead – marketing-speak for a shoe which can be used for a wide variety of sports and therefore is more than adequate for all but the most specialist of athletes.

Confused? Don't be. Sports-shoe design is big business and the manufacturers spend millions on modifying and remodifying the range of styles on offer, mainly, it must be said, to guarantee increased sales from what have become important fashion accessories. In 1990 Nike had 300 models worldwide, with 900 different styles, Reebok planned 250 new designs on top of their 175 existing models in 450 colours, and both Adidas and LA Gear had about 500 styles each. It has also been estimated that brand loyalty determines as much as 70 per cent of all repeat sales of training shoes, and that almost half the prospective customers have chosen the exact model of shoe before setting foot in a shop. A triumph for the seductive TV ad.

However, never feel pressurized into buying anything you're not 100 per cent satisfied with. Trainers are not cheap, and if they're not fitted properly, it's not only your body at risk but your bank balance.

The Bench

Steps, blocks, platforms, crates, BenchStep 2000, BodyBoard, Aerobic-Stair, Snap Step, SuperStep, Nextstep, Step Box, Instep, The Step, FitStep, A. S. Box. Call it what you like, a bench by any other name will make you sweat. And when it comes down to it, there are only really two types on offer – those you pay for and those you don't.

For instance, noting that one American programme used benches evolved from the design of milk crates, enterprising instructors from one club reportedly came to an arrangement with their local dairy and conducted their step classes quite successfully on the milk crates supplied. However, such crates are quite high for the beginner to work on, do not allow for any travelling steps because the surface is fairly small, and may not be sturdy enough for you. So in that case, turn to the hammer and nails. Yes, DIY fiend or not, creating your own bench out of wood may take you an hour or two, but it isn't difficult and it will ensure that it's exactly the right dimensions for you — and save you a lot of money.

You should be aiming at ½-inch (12mm) plywood for the main body of the bench, screwed and glued with wood on to an inner frame made from 1¼-inch-square (33mm²) strips of ply. (This frame will add strength, and will also help spread the load when you're working out so that it doesn't dig into your carpet.) The stepping surface should be about 14 inches (35cm) wide and between 36 and 48 inches (90 and 120cm) long, with a diagonal cross support screwed underneath to stop the wood flexing when you step up. The sides should then range in height from 4 to 8 inches (10 to 20cm), depending on your level of fitness and experience. Add a rubber car mat to the top to make the surface as non-slip as possible, and that's it. You have your bench, and

no more excuses.

And if you do get hooked, you can always buy a 'proper' bench later on. Since Connie Williams first convinced her Atlanta club to construct those three-man wooden monsters back in 1987, step technology has taken huge strides. Benches are available in moulded, high-molecular HDPE, polypropylene and high-density polyethylene (plastic, in other words). These terms are meaningless to most people, and wading through the glossy brochures can be a little daunting, especially when the all-important height of the bench seems almost a side issue when surrounded by the various load capacities, dimensions, anti-skid devices, total weight, portability . . . There's no substitute for trying them out in the shop to find the one with which you feel most comfortable.

Brand names aside, though, there's only one choice you really need to make and that's whether you go for a bench which has an adjustable height or one where the height is fixed — the latter usually being the cheapest option. And then you might like to look at the bench's length so that you can get the maximum amount of travelling steps into your routine. Stepping on a postage stamp can be very frustrating after a while. In reality, though, the selection at your local sports shop will probably determine your purchase,

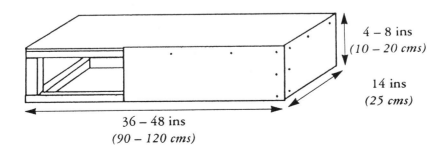

4 – 8 ins
(10 – 20 cms)

14 ins
(25 cms)

36 – 48 ins
(90 – 120 cms)

since in my experience retailers tend to stock just one brand. If you want alternatives, read through the small ads of any fitness magazine – like *Shape* or *Health & Fitness* – and go direct to the distributors. The good news is that more and more benches are coming on the market all the time, prices are coming down, and you can now pick one up for about the price of a pair of jeans.

The Sound of Step

And so to music, the main factor which can motivate you or leave you flagging within seconds of starting. For whether it's a hoedown or salsa that really gets you moving, the music's there for one reason and one reason only: to keep you working in time – something made abundantly clear after seeing two partially deaf women stepping out to a good strong rhythm.

When it comes to benchwork, the tempo is regular and easy – approximately 120 beats per minute or two beats per second – and far fewer than the lung-busting 130–160 bpm common in more conventional aerobic routines. Let's face it, it would be nigh on impossible to sustain a good step workout for any length of time at that sort of tempo, and it would also be dangerous. If you didn't fall off, you'd certainly not have time

to make your moves. Benchwork is not about frenetic activity but sheer hard work, and the tempo of your routine reflects this fact.

So what do you do if you're stepping at home? You can't exactly switch on the radio and march away to whatever's playing, and no one album is going to be appropriate from start to finish – although many 'rave' albums come close. Moreover, thumbing through old favourites which have the 120 bpm-tempo – such as Michael Jackson's 'Billy Jean', or 'Suicide Blonde' by INXS, 'Good Vibrations' by Markie Mark or maybe C & C Music Factory's 'Things that Make You Go HMMM', – with a view to making up your own tape would be great – if only it wasn't illegal. What you can do, though, is turn to those small ads at the back of fitness magazines, because there are always good step compilations on offer – even good enough to listen to for pleasure, as long as your feet don't instinctively start marching up and down as soon as the music starts.

When it comes down to it, you can spend as much or as little as you want when kitting up for a benchwork routine. I have a selection of leggings and support tops because I can't be bothered washing them out every other night. But if you are strapped for cash at the moment, think about your feet first, and work upward from there.

chapter four

Watch Your Step

The Dos and Don'ts of Benchwork

IT WOULD BE nice to view benchwork as just another fun aerobic workout, and one where your body magically burns off all its excess fat, your muscles mysteriously tone themselves up and all you have to do is walk away at the end of it with a totally transformed physique. Except, of course, that benchwork is not just your average aerobic workout – invigorating, yes, and able to give your heart and lungs a thorough going-over, but control is the key word when it comes to this form of exercise, and it should not be approached lightly.

The last thing anybody wants to do is read through a boring old list of dos and don'ts when you've got your music, you've got your bench and you're waiting there ready for action. But in many ways benchwork is more like a standing conditioning workout than anything else, a programme in which you work your body through specific movements to achieve the desired tone and shape. And you really do need to concentrate hard on your posture and technique all the time to ensure that you don't ask the impossible of your body and so risk injury.

So, while step training has been designed to reduce the stresses and strains on your body as much as possible, its safety and effectiveness are dependent on you. And if you ignore the basic principles behind the programme, you are only asking for trouble. A 100 per cent 'safe' form of exercise simply does not exist. All you can do is inform yourself about any potential dangers and how best to avoid them. And as always, if you are very unfit, very overweight, pregnant or getting on a bit, or have any medical history of problems with your heart, blood pressure, lungs or any combination of the above – be careful. And if you do experience any discomfort – stop. Simple really.

1. **Good posture is at the heart of good stepping and if you get this right, everything else in the programme will fall into place naturally.**

So, before going any further, stand in front of a full-length mirror and practise standing up straight! Indeed, if you can work out in front of a mirror, so much the better because you can then keep an eagle eye on the slightest hint of bad technique and correct it accordingly.

Stand with your feet a little apart, with your neck and shoulders relaxed, knees 'soft' — in other words, don't straighten them rigidly, or 'lock out' the joint — and stomach muscles pulled in tight. You should never arch your back while stepping, so drop those buttocks a little by tilting your pelvis forward.

Now imagine that someone has attached a piece of string to the top of your head and is pulling it gently upward, lifting your upper body out of your hips. This is the posture you should be aiming at whilst stepping — a strong stance, and a balanced one, taking the pressure off your hips and knees through the control of your upper body. Approach your bench.

2. **Place your right foot slowly on your bench, remembering the three 'F's — *full foot flat* — and leading up through your heel — NOT bouncing up on to the ball of your foot.**

You want your footing to be as stable as possible, to reduce the stress on your ankles and calves. If you allow your heel to hang over the back edge, you not only throw out your balance but increase the amount of pressure on your lower leg. Glance down at regular intervals to ensure that your footing is correct.

3. **There should be a gentle diagonal running from the left heel upwards to the back of your head when you step up. Think of that person pulling you upwards with that piece of string and allow your body to follow the**

top of your head in a natural, uplifted movement. Keep your chest raised and stomach muscles strong to help support your back and resist the force of gravity.

Stooping forward from the waist at an exaggerated angle may put unnecessary strain on the lower back and thus lead to problems.

4. **Keep the heel of your supporting leg pressed down firmly as you bring the left foot up to join it. If you place your hand just under your buttocks, the back of your thigh should feel tense and flexed. Make sure that you achieve this feeling every time you are supported on one foot — be it in a knee lift, leg curl, whatever — so that you ensure you are pushing downward through your heel all the time.**

This will not only help tone up your buttocks and hamstrings but will also safeguard against unnecessary stress on your ankles, knees and calves.

5. **Stand tall when you are on the bench. Your knees should be 'soft' but not bent.**

There are a lot of muscles in your knee, and all need to be extended when you step up so that they are allowed to work through the full range of their motion. So stand tall — but don't lock them out rigidly.

6. **Step off the platform with your right foot, again keeping that same strong body position with your chest well lifted so that you resist the force of gravity pulling you down and don't just collapse off the back. You want to cushion your joints as much as possible, so lead downward with the ball of your foot, and let the heel simply melt down into the floor.**

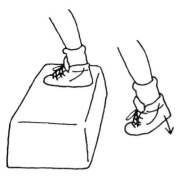

The ball of the foot lands first, followed by the heel

Although this action only takes a third of the energy of stepping up (according to the ACSM *Guidelines*), it is this downward movement off the bench which exerts the greatest force on the joints. It therefore stands to reason that you should try to soften the impact as much as possible.

According to a recent article by Tony Lycholat in *Health & Fitness* magazine about Step Reebok, a delayed muscle soreness in the calves is not unusual after the first step training session, and is usually because of an uneven loading on the calf muscles when stepping down. The good news is, however, that this soreness does disperse once your body has become used to the step movement – I experienced some next-day stiffness first time round, but have never had a problem with this since.

Nevertheless, to gauge your susceptibility to this type of problem, Lycholat goes on to provide a test to check what he calls your 'calf risk'. Take your shoes off and stand with your back to a wall. Keeping your heels firmly planted on the floor, raise the ball of each foot in turn while a friend sees if he or she can ease two fingers in the gap left underneath. If this isn't possible, you lack flexibility in your calves and should gradually ease them out with a series of different stretches to this area. It's probably advisable to seek professional help here.

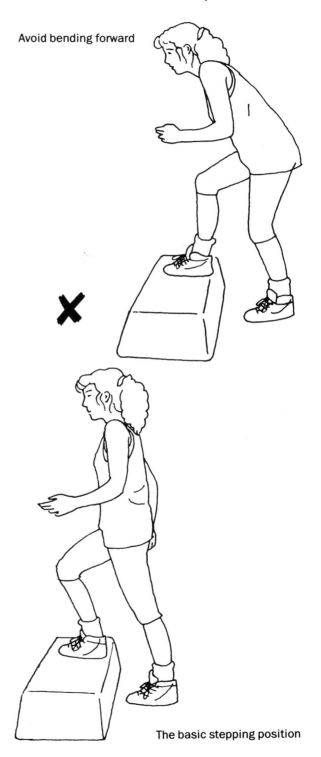

Avoid bending forward

The basic stepping position

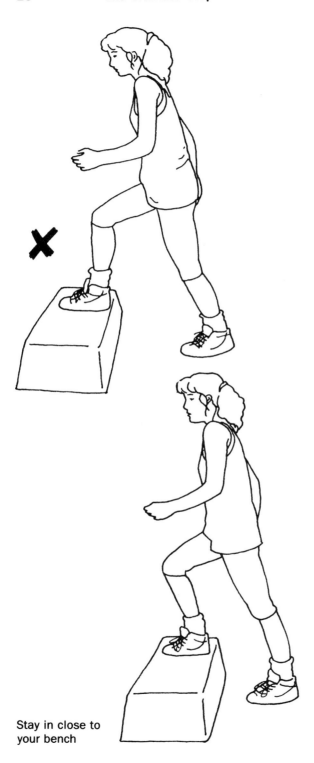

X

Stay in close to
your bench

7. Keep your feet in close to your bench when stepping down to maintain the proper body alignment. Step off too far backwards and you'll tend to lean forward too much.

8. Stamping is out! You should hardly make a sound when stepping up or down.

Marching heavily on the bench when you step up and thumping down again on the floor when you descend means that you're not cushioning your joints properly and so increasing the risk of injury.

9. No matter what your height, no matter how practised at benchwork you are, no matter what your fitness level, you should never step up so high that your knees are flexed more than 90 degrees.

Flex them more than this and you are not only putting them under unnecessary stress, but you are also running the risk of compromising your posture since you will necessarily bend too far forward to achieve the movement and so put undue pressure on your lower back. If you want to increase the cardiorespiratory demand of your workout once you have started working at eight inches, extend the length of your routine.

10. Don't twist your knees! Try and make sure that you always keep the knee of your supporting leg in line with your ankle.

11. When you start stepping, always balance the work done on each side of the body by regularly changing the leading leg – in other words, the leg which you step up with.

12. Even if you start to make up your own steps and routines, *never* step forward off your board as you would if simply going down a flight of stairs.

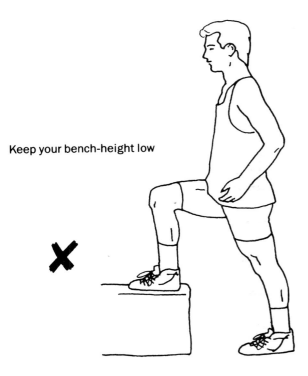

Keep your bench-height low

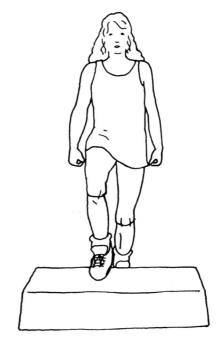

Keep your knee and ankle in line

To protect the joints, always descend backwards or sideways — you can control the movement much better and so land more softly, cushioning yourself in the process.

13. **Execute every step and leg movement in a controlled manner, working against your own resistance all the time and isolating and focusing on the muscles in question.**

14. **Drink lots of fluid, before, during and after your workout. You will sweat a lot when step training and it's important to replenish your reserves to prevent dehydration (see p.101).**

15. **And last, but by no means least, be careful when carrying your bench around the room.**

Having just completed one of the most vigorous aerobic workouts, and having toned your muscles up beautifully, it would be a shame to fall at the very last hurdle by twisting something

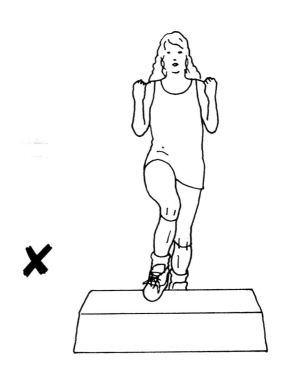

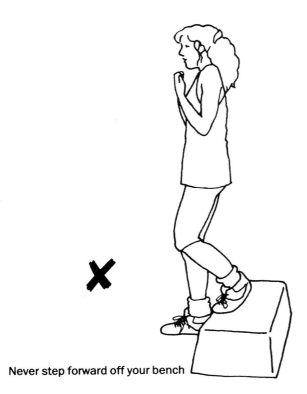

Never step forward off your bench

when putting your bench away. So be sensible. Bend your knees when picking it up and don't hold the platform out in front of you at arm's length when carrying it around.

So do it right! The good news is that reports of injury through benchwork are few and far between, and those that have occurred were mainly due to people trying to step up on to benches which are too high for them. As I said at the start, there is no such thing as a totally safe fitness programme and, no matter how carefully you work, there is still a chance that you may pull a muscle or twist a joint. But the fact of the matter is that the vast majority of people stepping do so without any ill effects whatsoever, making benchwork not only an effective, time-efficient training programme, but also a successful one from the safety angle. And the less time you spend nursing sore muscles, the more time you have to get fit.

chapter five

Warming Up

The First Step to Fitness

ENTION THE WORD 'warm-up' to most people, and painful memories of jogging round the school sports field on a frosty winter's morning come flooding back. But it can be a far less daunting experience than that — even marching round the room a few times or bopping along to the radio will do — as long as you mobilize and ease out both upper and lower body with the exercises listed in this chapter. What you're aiming at is simply to get your heart rate going so that your system is primed and ready for action (see Appendix 1), and literally warm your body up, loosening up your joints and easing our your muscles. Why? To help lessen the effect on your body's soft tissue of the demanding workout you're about to do — not to mention making the actual stepping as productive a quarter- or half-hour session as possible. It'll take at least seven or eight minutes to warm your body up — more like ten or twelve if it's cold or first thing in the morning — so let it. A few minutes' patience

at this end could well prevent a painful injury later on.

Loosen Up

Of course, it may well be the first time that you have used a certain muscle in a long time — in fact, it may be the first time ever, and you'll probably feel sore with even the mildest of stretches. So take it easy and never force anything. No shaking limbs, no stress or strain. Just nice, relaxed movements. And if at any time you feel a sharp pain or any obvious discomfort, stop immediately.

Stretching a Point

A few things to think about when approaching your stretches.

1. **Make sure that you have warmed your body up first before going into any stretch.**

Some people like to wear a sweatshirt at the start of their workout – especially in winter.

2. Ease in and out of the positions as if you're doing them in slow motion.

If a muscle or tendon is suddenly put under stress it will automatically contract in order to protect itself by using its so-called 'stretch reflex'. Sneak up on the muscle instead. Move into position bit by bit, easing gently into the stretch and then hold it there until the muscle has got used to the tension. After about ten seconds you'll feel this tension drain away as the muscle returns to its normal length.

3. Breathe! Take a deep breath in and exhale when you move into a stretch, breathing normally once you're in position.

Your body will relax more and make the action more effective.

4. Don't bounce!

Momentum – even in movements like touching your toes – can easily push a muscle or joint too far.

5. Always balance the stretches.

Whatever you do on one side, do on the other too. Most people tend to be slightly more flexible on one side than on the other so try to concentrate a little more on your worse side to balance up your body.

Of course, the great thing about stretching is that you can see results almost immediately, because even if you are fairly stiff to begin with and face the prospect of several weeks' practice before you gain any real degree of flexibility, by the end of any stretching session you will be able to move all your limbs that little bit more freely and so really feel the benefits. However, if you are new to exercising, you might find it easier to do all the stretches below in isolation.

The Bench Warm-up

So put some music on to get you in the mood, take a quick sip of water, a deep breath, relax – and approach your bench ready to begin.

1. **Stand facing the long side of your bench, with your feet hip-width apart, toes pointing outward a little and knees relaxed. Think about that piece of string attached to the top of your head, pulling you gently upward and lengthening your spine. Suck your stomach in, tilt your pelvis slightly forward and bend your knees as you inhale, drawing your arms out to either side of you and upward above your head in a wide arc, straightening your knees again as you go. Hold it briefly and exhale, bringing your arms down to your sides again before repeating this all again – giving your body a good boost of oxygen before you start.**

   Repeat 3 times

2. **Now bring your feet together and begin marching on the spot, pumping your arms – that is, working them backward and forward with your hands loosely clenched, as if you are running – and making sure that the ball of your foot hits the ground first with each step before rolling down into your heel. Keep your knees soft and upper body relaxed.**

   Repeat for 16 beats

3. **This time take a step forward on the floor with your right foot, bringing your left up beside it, and then a step back with your right, your left following suit once again, marching your body gently into the rhythm of benchwork.**

   Repeat 16 times

4. **Now draw your feet apart until they are about hip width from each other and continue marching vigorously as before. Pick**

those knees up and pump those arms —
even though it may feel a little awkward
to begin with!

Repeat 16 times

5. Still keeping your feet apart, bring your
hands on to your hips and gently start bending your knees up and down in an easy squat
in time to the music, keeping your back nice
and straight, stomach pulled in with a pelvic
tilt and making sure that your knees travel
over your toes. Never squat down so far that
there is less than a 90-degree angle at your
knee, and don't lock them out — that is, don't
straighten them completely — as you come
up.

Repeat 8 times

6. With every two squats, gently look over
slightly to your right and then back to the
centre again, over to your left for the count
of two and back to the centre again in one
continuous movement. Take care never to
yank your neck or drop your chin forward or
backward as you turn, and keep your shoulders and arms relaxed, letting your jaw drop
a little if you like. Your upper body should
remain facing the front all the time.

Repeat 8 times

Always be careful with your neck. It is probably the last thing you think of warming up
but ironically it is the one area where tension
is most likely to build up, since it is only when
you are asleep that it is not actually working.
Twist it accidentally, though, and you'll soon
notice how much you do use it — so start as
you mean to go on and warm it up first of all.

7. Return your head to the centre and, still
squatting gently up and down, start circling
your right shoulder backwards in time to the
music, increasing the movement after eight

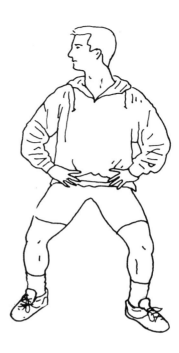

The wide squat, head to the right

so that you begin circling your right elbow
back at the same time and then, after eight
more, extending the movement again so that
you circle your right arm back a further eight
times.

Repeat on the left

8. Now start marching on the spot once again,
keeping your feet apart and toes pointing
outward, pumping your arms as if you were
running. Don't be lazy! Lift up those knees
and really prepare those thighs and buttocks
for the work they are about to do.

Repeat for 16 beats

9. Bring your feet together and continue
marching on the spot, pumping your arms
vigorously and lifting up those knees.

Repeat for 16 beats

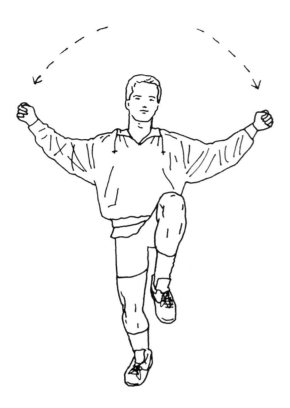

Knee lift — with lateral pull-down

10. Continue pumping your arms, but this time tap your toes gently on top of your bench with alternate feet, keeping the knee of your supporting leg soft all the time. You are preparing your hips, buttocks and thighs for actually stepping up on to your platform.
Repeat for 16 beats

11. Now lift each knee up even further, touching it with both hands as you bring it as near to waist height as you can manage. Don't overstretch yourself — but certainly don't fall asleep — and remember to keep your supporting leg soft all the time, with your heel pushed down firmly into the ground.
Alternate left and right 8 times

12. Reach out in front of you with both hands and, every time you lift a knee, pull both arms back in a big arc at your sides, increasing the amount of work in your heart and lungs whilst mobilizing your upper body. Then stretch your arms above your head and repeat the movement, pulling both arms downward this time, but resisting the action all the way.
Repeat 8 times pulling backward,
8 times pulling downward,
8 times pulling backward and
finally 8 pulling downward

13. To increase the work in your hips, buttocks and thighs, now do a set of four knee lifts with your right leg, four knee lifts with your left, still raising them up so that you can touch them with both hands at about waist height.
Do 6 sets of 4 on alternate legs
before returning to 8 single knee lifts

14. Start marching on the spot again, pumping your arms vigorously and picking your knees up, before tapping on top of your bench with your toes again.
Repeat for 16 beats

15. Shoulder Stretch
It's time to stretch out those shoulders, so bring your left arm up and across the body at shoulder height, keeping the elbow soft but easing out the shoulder joint a fraction by pressing your raised arm gently into your body with your right hand. As always, keep your upper body relaxed and neck and spine lengthened. Gently ease out of the position.
Hold for about 10 seconds and
repeat on the other side

16. Triceps Stretch
Raise your left arm above your head and,

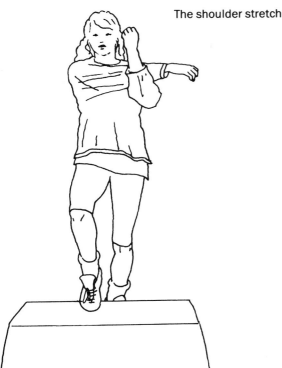

The shoulder stretch

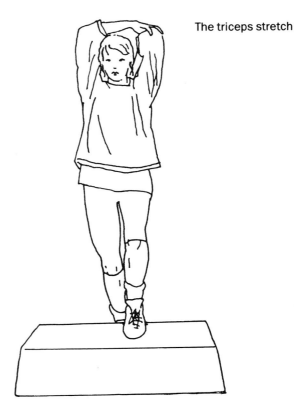

The triceps stretch

keeping your elbow pointing straight up to the ceiling, drop your left hand down behind your head so that it is resting between your shoulder blades. Now hold on to your left arm just above your elbow with your right hand and gently pull it inward towards your head so that you feel a stretching in the upper part of your raised arm. Gently ease out of the position.

Hold for about 10 seconds and
repeat on the other side

17. Moving down the body, it's time to begin working the thighs and buttocks a little more. So, place your hands on your hips and stand with your feet about a foot and a half apart — or at a comfortable distance from each other — toes pointing slightly outward, and bend your knees into an easy squat

keeping your stomach and buttocks tucked in. Start pushing from side to side so that you feel a slight tension in the inside of the thighs. Your knees should be relaxed at all times; be careful not to arch your back.

Repeat 16 times

18. Now turn your left foot to face the front and hold that position over to your right for about 16 beats, then swap sides and hold once more.

19. It's now the turn of the calves, so hold that easy squat in the centre, checking your posture in the mirror to make sure that your stomach is pulled in and pelvis tilted slightly forward, and raise alternate heels.

Continue this throughout the next two
upper-body stretches

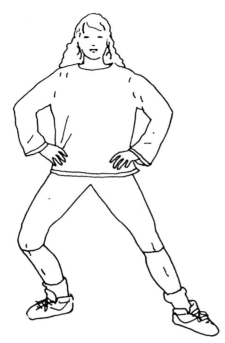

Side-to-side push, feet apart

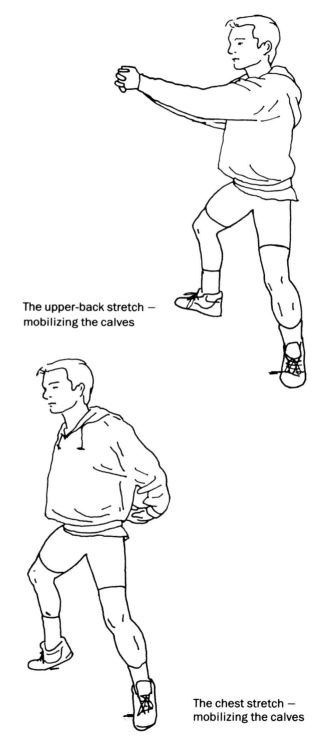

The upper-back stretch —
mobilizing the calves

20. Upper-back Stretch

With your lower body now relatively station-
ary, it is an excellent time to begin stretching
your top half. Lock your fingers together and
raise your hands in front of you at shoulder
height as if you were holding an elongated
beach ball. This is to ensure that you never
lock out your elbow joints and so put them
under stress. Inhale and then exhale so that
you feel a mild tension pulling your shoulder
blades apart.

*Hold for about 10 seconds
and gently ease out of the stretch*

21. Chest Stretch

Still working your calf muscles, clasp your
hands behind the small of your back, fingers interlocked as before, your elbows
always soft, and gently try to push your

The chest stretch —
mobilizing the calves

shoulders backwards so that your shoulder blades meet in the middle. Keep your chest up and don't arch your back.

Hold for about 10 seconds and gently ease out of the stretch

22. Place your hands on your hips once more and, with your feet planted firmly on the ground, start pushing your whole body from side to side for a few beats. Then, lowering your hands on to the fronts of your thighs and bending forward from the hips a little with a good straight back, rock gently each way but this time lift your toes off the floor while your heels remain firmly planted. As always, keep your stomach pulled in and don't arch your back.

Repeat 16 times

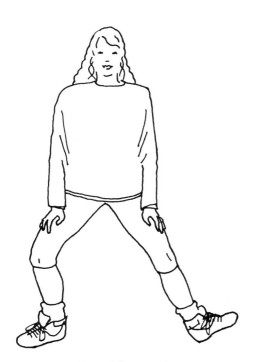

Rock from side to side, raising your toes

From here it is easy to move into two stretching movements, one for the front of the thighs and hips, and one for the calves — both movements stemming from the same basic position.

23. **Stretching Out the Thighs and Hips**
Stand with your feet about twice hip-width apart in an easy squat, and turn your whole body to the left so that your left knee is directly over your left ankle. Your right heel should be off the floor behind you with the right knee slightly bent, and both feet should be pointing straight ahead. Tuck in your stomach and draw your pelvis slightly forward until you feel a stretching sensation down the front of your right thigh. Both arms should be extended at chest height in front of you for balance.

Now, keeping your back upright, bend your left knee so that your right is lowered towards the floor — but never touches it — and then raise yourself again, stretching out the right thigh and hips as you do so. Pull back with both arms as you lower yourself and reach forward again as you return to your starting position. If at any point you feel any undue pressure on your left knee or find the movement awkward, try the quadriceps stretch on p82 instead.

Repeat 8 times

24. **Calf Stretch**
From here, draw your right foot in towards your left a little, still keeping both feet pointing straight in front of you, but this time gently lower your right heel on to the floor so that you feel a gentle stretch down your right calf.

Repeat 8 times

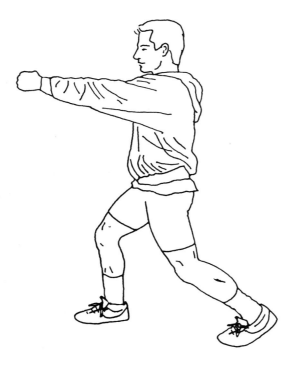

Both the thigh and hip stretch and calf stretch can be increased when you become more flexible by placing your front foot flat on top of the bench. Nevertheless, in both cases still make sure that your knee is placed directly over your ankle, not pushed forward.

25. Stomach and Buttocks Squeeze
Gently twist round again so that you are facing your bench, holding the wide squat, hands on thighs, with a full body lean so that your body weight is supported on your thighs. Suck in your stomach and buttocks in an exaggerated pelvic tilt, squeezing for all you're worth and rounding your back gently as you do so. Hold it briefly and relax, pressing your buttocks backward over your heels as you straighten out your lower back.

Repeat 4 times

26. Turn to your right and repeat numbers 23, 24 and 25 on the other side.

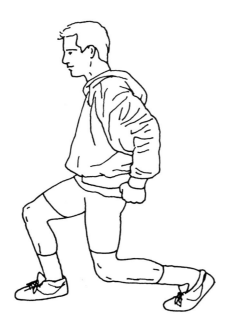

The thigh and hip stretch

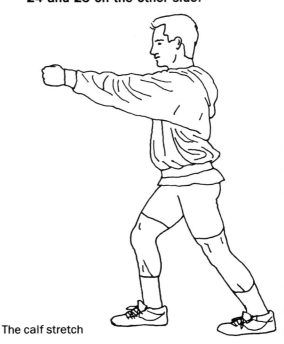

The calf stretch

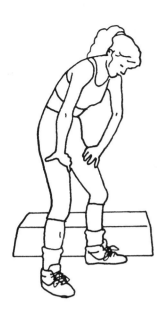

27. Slowly begin marching on the spot again, this time pumping your arms by your sides to get the circulation going again.

    Repeat 16 times

28. Hamstring Stretch

    Keeping your hips high and head and neck in line with your spine, carefully place the flexed heel of your right foot in the centre of your platform and bend the supporting leg. Your left foot should be pointing straight ahead of you. Your upper body will naturally lean forward until you feel a gentle stretch in the back of your thigh and you will probably want to support yourself with your arms. Do not push down on the raised leg — your knees can only straighten so far! This stretch also eases out the neck, spine, buttocks and — as you can probably feel — calf muscles.

    Hold for at least 15 seconds — 5 with the foot flexed, 5 slowly pushing the foot flat on to the bench and 5 gently flexing the foot again

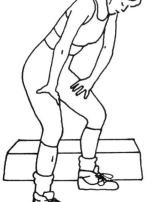

The stomach and buttocks squeeze

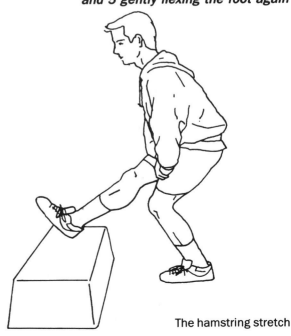

The hamstring stretch

29. Lower Calf Stretch

From that position, place your raised foot flat on the bench, shift your weight forward and carefully draw your back foot inward. Now bend both knees a little by lowering yourself downward over your back heel until you feel a gentle stretch in your lower calf there. Keep your upper body relaxed and in line, and support yourself by placing both hands on the raised thigh.

Hold for about 10 seconds

Remember to bend both knees as you ease yourself out of the stretch and curl your upper body towards the ceiling, vertebra by vertebra, so that you protect your spine.

Repeat numbers 28 and 29 on the left

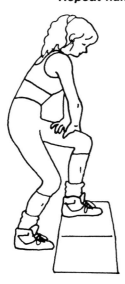

The lower calf stretch

Take care with these stretches if you have a history of lower-back problems. In this case, do exactly the same movements but without propping your foot up on the bench, still being very careful not to twist or jerk your spine in any way, and making doubly sure that your hips are kept high and supporting leg bent throughout.

30. Having slowed the pace down slightly during the preceding stretches, there is a chance that your body might have begun to cool down, so it's time to get your system going in a way which will lead you into the step routine to come.

a. Begin tapping your toes on top of your bench with alternate feet — down, tap, down, tap — starting with your right, and pump your arms vigorously once more.

b. After eight beats, actually step up on to the bench with your right foot, making sure that the whole of your trainer is on the platform — *including* your heel (it's amazing how many people think that their feet end at their insteps) — and march on the top for eight more beats, working your arms all the time.

c. Then step back off your bench, again with your right, rolling through your foot from the ball to the heel as you land so that you cushion yourself on the way down and so protect your joints. Again march it out, this time on the floor, for eight beats.

d. Step up again with your right foot, but this time only march on top for four beats before stepping back off again, to march to the count of four on the floor.

Repeat

e. And for the final set, step up with your right, bringing your left foot up to follow it, and then immediately step down again with your right, your left once more in hot pursuit.

Repeat 4 times
Repeat 30a–e twice
and then continue marching on the spot
before changing sides

Whether you realize it or not, you have just performed the basic up-up-down-down step which lies at the heart of all benchwork programmes. It's a very simple action, focusing the work on the thighs and buttocks, but remember — even this most basic of movements repeated for a quarter of an hour on alternate sides can burn up a surprising amount of calories. So stand tall, lift yourself upward from your head and lead through your heels to perfect your technique and safeguard against any chances of injury later on.

chapter six

Working Out

The First-timer's Guide to Stepping

NOBODY LIKES TO be thought of as a beginner. It means that you've got a lot to learn, that you've got to practise . . . in short, it means all those things you really don't want to think about once you've finally decided to take the plunge and get fit. However, *anyone* who has never stepped before, from the fittest marathon runner to the champion telly addict, is considered a benchwork beginner – a first-timer. Step is a great leveller.

Stepping Out

This first group of steps will introduce you to the exercises which form the basis of all benchwork programmes. Master these, and you will march your way through any number of complicated step patterns later on. They all work the bench face-on – in other words, the long side of your bench is in front of you. So, providing your full foot is supported and you have enough space to stretch your arms out comfortably at your sides, there

is nothing to stop you trying out this first benchwork routine at the bottom of a flight of stairs.

If at any time you get lost or find it difficult to co-ordinate both parts of the body at the same time, forget about your arms and just keep your hands on your hips. At this stage, it is far more important to get your legs working automatically than worry about which arm should be doing what and when. After all, your legs account for at least 85 per cent of the energy cost of stepping – a good incentive to get your footwork right if ever there was one.

You should treat the opening movements as a practice session and repeat every one about eight times on each side, concentrating on technique at every stage and reading through Chapter Four just once more to make sure that all the dos and don'ts really have sunk in. Benchwork is all about control and correct execution. Get that right, and the heavy breathing will follow all too soon.

Take a sip of water so that your system is fully topped up and begin by marching on the spot in time to the music behind your bench, keeping your upper body relaxed and letting your arms swing loosely by your sides. Then start stepping up and down leading with your right leg, really pushing down through your heels, lifting up out of your hips and pumping your arms a bit more vigorously as if you were running.

Changing the Leading Leg – The Tap Down

After eight or so steps, change your leading leg by *tapping down* – the basic step which ensures you work both sides of your body evenly. So step backwards off your bench with your right foot as usual, but this time, as soon as the ball of your left foot touches the floor – or *taps down* – bring it straight back up on to the bench again and step up on to it. Your left foot is now leading with your right foot following. In other words, simply tap the ground with your left foot, rather than putting all your weight on to it, and begin stepping with it as normal.

Carry on leading with your left leg, again concentrating on your technique, and then tap down with the right this time so that you are back on to your right once more. Carry on pumping your arms vigorously by your sides.

Alternate Tap Down

You can develop this idea of changing the leading leg until you tap down after every step. So, warm up into the alternate tap down by stepping up and down as normal for eight steps leading with your right, before tapping down and doing eight on your left. Tap down and return to your right for just four steps this time before tapping down and repeating this on the other side. Now tap down and do doubles on each side, then singles so that you tap down every time your trailing foot hits the ground. In this way, you are tapping down on alternate feet. Simple.

Spend the next couple of minutes working on this until you have it off pat and can tap down in your sleep.

Changing the Leading Leg – The Tap Up

Now, still pumping your arms, change your tapping down to a tap *up* – exactly the same step, but this time you are tapping *on top* of the bench instead of on the floor, the tapping foot hitting the top and stepping straight back off again in order to change the leading leg once again.

Alternate Tap Up

Similarly, build into the alternate tap up in exactly the same way you did for the tap down, tapping up after eight steps on each side, after every four, every two and finally after every step so that you are continually changing the leading leg and working each side evenly. Again, practice makes perfect – so do!

The Knee Lift

The tap up is an important step to master because several other moves develop out of it. The most simple is the knee lift, although for some reason many first-timers do seem to find problems here and end up with their feet going all over the place, never again quite managing to catch up. If this happens to you, you're thinking too much!

Start stepping normally with your right leg, tapping up on top of the bench after about four steps and continue with this pattern on the left, tapping up after four again until you've really

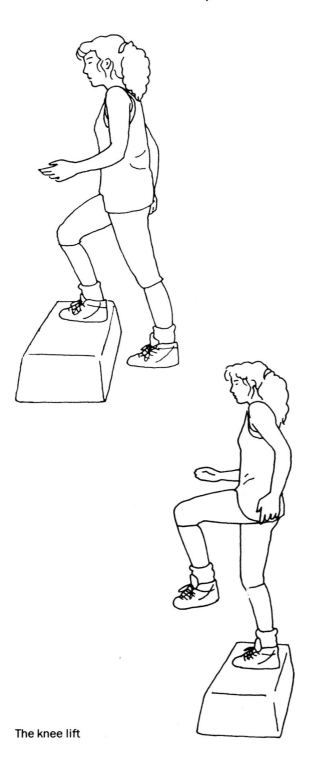

The knee lift

got into the rhythm of it. Let the beat of your music carry you along and keep you balanced.

This time, instead of tapping the bench each time, draw your leg straight up into a knee lift and down to the ground again before continuing to step as normal. Don't tap up *then* do a knee lift. Don't move beautifully into a knee lift and lose it at the last minute by only lowering your foot as far as your bench. It's just straight up and straight down to the floor again, without stopping halfway to enjoy the view.

Alternate Knee Lifts

Having mastered the basic action, it is time to increase the intensity of the exercise by doing a knee lift every time you step up on to the bench. Again, don't think about it too much and, as you've just practised with the alternate tap up and tap down, build into the alternate knee lift from eights down to singles so that your leading leg changes every time.

Leg Curls

While the knee lift mainly works the front of the thigh and hip, leg curls balance that out by focusing on the back of the thigh — the hamstring.

Start stepping as before, leading with your right leg, and tap up after every four steps. Now substitute a leg curl for each tap up by drawing your heel up towards your buttocks. Find the contraction as your foot rises and squeeze it briefly before relaxing it again as your foot steps down on to the floor once more. You might like to place your hand behind your thigh and feel the muscles work. But whatever you do, keep the supporting leg firmly planted, your thighs fairly close together and your hips square. Don't arch your back, and lead up through your chest

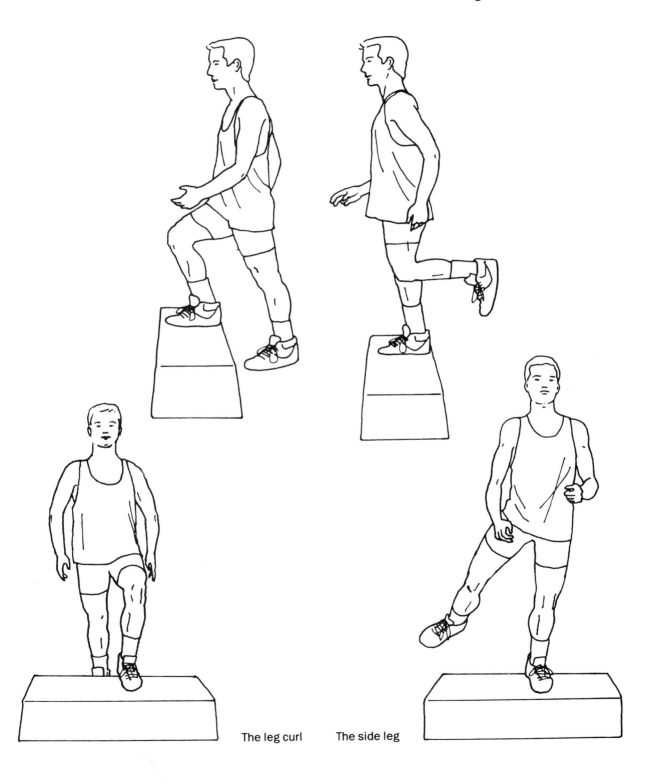

The leg curl   The side leg

– just keep your stomach pulled in and really make those hamstrings work.

Continue stepping normally for four more steps and then curl the other foot back – squeezing all the time – to change the leading leg. Practise the move until you've got it off pat.

Side Leg

Now on to the side leg, a small, controlled, squeezing movement in which you raise the leg straight out to the side with the foot flexed and pointing to the front – not up towards the ceiling as you would if doing a side kick when dancing. Keep your hips square as you push the leg outward and remember – it is not the height you raise it that counts, but the amount you squeeze your buttocks which determines how toned and pert your backside becomes. So keep the movement low and the heel of the supporting leg well pressed down – and watch how well your buttocks shape up!

As with the knee lifts, you can then practise doing both leg curls and side legs continuously on alternate sides so that the buttocks and thighs get a thorough workout.

The V-Step

A slightly different movement which also focuses on the buttocks and inner thigh muscles is the wide-marching V-step. So return to the straight step leading with your right foot and this time, instead of keeping your feet at a natural distance from each other, stride out so that they end up pointing outward at either end of the platform. Step back down, bringing your feet together again on the floor – hence the V-shape – and repeat this open–close movement.

Tap down with your left foot and continue practising this movement on the other side.

The Wide Step

To intensify this, step *down* with your feet in a wide stance as well so that you work the muscles doubly hard. Ungainly and a bit robotic though this feels when you first start, it never allows the buttocks to relax, so tap down once again and begin working with the right leg, concentrating on the muscles you want to contract before tapping down to repeat this on the left.

Then, as for all the other movements so far, start tapping down after each side. Familiarity is what you are aiming at for the moment, familiarity with the bench itself and the type of moves involved so that you build your confidence whilst perfecting your technique.

The Arms

It is time to bring in some basic arm movements. But remember – whatever arm exercises you do and whether you are familiar with them or not, control is what you are aiming for. There is no point in just going through the motions. Work against your own resistance and really try to feel the muscles contracting. Although all the arm movements in this chapter remain below shoulder height, don't be surprised at the difference they seem to make to the intensity of the routine.

You might like to practise all the following arm movements at half-speed away from your bench to begin with, taking four counts to complete each until you are quite sure about the action. Then approach your bench and start stepping normally before leading into the alternate tap down. Introduce each arm movement in turn to the four-beat count before increasing your arm speed to two-count movements.

The Bicep Curl

The first and simplest arm exercise to incorporate is the bicep curl, an exercise common to all toning classes and familiar to anyone who's ever watched a Popeye cartoon.

Bring both arms down to your sides, with your palms facing your outer thighs, hands lightly clenched and elbows close into your waist. Keeping your shoulders relaxed and upper arms still, take the lock off your elbows and bend them *slightly* so that you find the greatest point of contraction. Hold it there for a few seconds so that you know what it feels like and what you should be aiming at every time you drop your hands into this position.

Then, the next time you step up on to the bench, curl both hands up towards your shoulders in a straight line so that the muscles are always under tension, adding a twisting movement to your forearms so that your hands end up facing your shoulders as your left foot lands on the bench. When you step down again, lower your hands to their starting position too, keeping your elbows tucked well into your sides and controlling the movement. (The twist is important because you want to make sure that you are using as much of the muscle as possible.) When stepping up and down like this, it is easy to rely on your body's momentum to swing your arms for you, although you won't tone your muscles this way.

Once you've got the bicep curl off pat, increase the pace so that you are working at the correct speed. On the count of one, begin the arm movement so that, as before, your hands are at shoulder height as you stand on top of the bench for the count of two. Then quickly drop your hands to your sides again for the count of three – still controlling the action, of course – and draw your hands upward once more on the

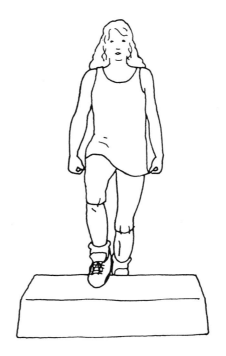

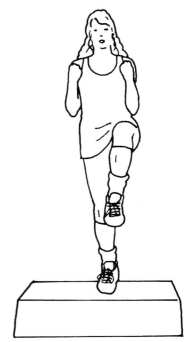

The bicep curl – with a knee lift

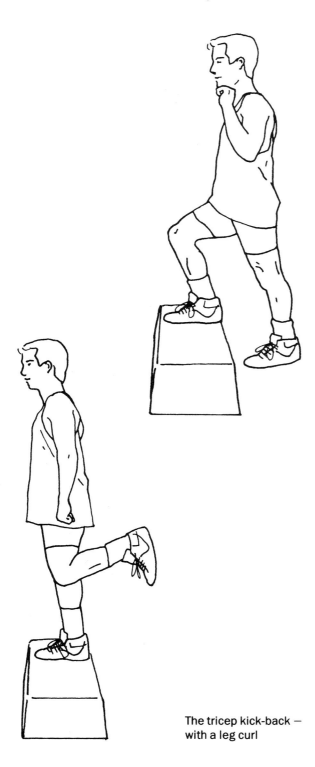

The tricep kick-back — with a leg curl

count of four as you stand with both feet on the floor, ready to begin the whole movement all over again.

It can seem confusing at first, trying to co-ordinate the correct bit of the arm movement with the correct bit of the step — and it doesn't *really* matter if you don't get it right anyway, as long as both are executed properly. But as a general rule of thumb, as long as you always begin both arm movement and step on the count of one, you'll find that they sit comfortably together, each complementing the other's motion so that your body action is always balanced.

The Tricep Kick-back

The body is all about balance — and there's no point having nice tight biceps if your arms are all saggy underneath, so the next exercise is one which works the triceps behind your upper arm.

With your elbows at your sides, bring both hands up towards your shoulders again, but this time with your palms facing away from you. Lightly clench your fists and drop them forward slightly as if you are holding on to the handlebars of a bicycle, and try to locate the muscles by contracting them a little. This isn't as easy as finding your biceps, so take a bit of time and really feel them, squeezing slightly before you do the full movement.

Now, the next time you step up, press *downward* through your arms, consciously contracting the triceps and using them alone to draw your hands down and very slightly round and towards the back of your body, with the elbow joints almost, but not quite, locked out. Squeeze the muscle, and slowly bring your hands back to the starting position as you step off the bench again, trying to keep your back straight, upper arms still and elbows tucked in throughout.

Repeat this whole movement, practising it until you get to know the muscle a little better and can isolate and squeeze it comfortably. Then continue the kick-back at normal speed as with the bicep curl above.

The Shoulders

And now to bring the shoulders into play with a couple of exercises which will start working the major muscles in this area.

Lat Raises

Bring both hands down in front of you, with your palms facing each other and arms slightly flexed. As you step up on to your platform with your right foot, lift your arms out to the sides and up to just above shoulder level, keeping the elbows high. It might help to imagine that your arms are being pulled outward and upward by your elbows so that you maintain the correct position throughout – and thus work the muscles in your shoulders and back properly.

Then, as you step off the bench once more, slowly lower your arms to the starting position, resisting the movement all the time. Concentrate on the action. If you're doing the exercise correctly, you should feel a tightening in the tops of your shoulders relatively quickly.

When you've mastered the movement, it's time to increase the pace so that you do one out-in movement with the arms as you step up on to the bench, and one as you step off it again, practising until you feel comfortable with it.

Upright Rows

To continue working this area, drop your hands down close together in front of you with your palms facing your pelvis, and pretend that you

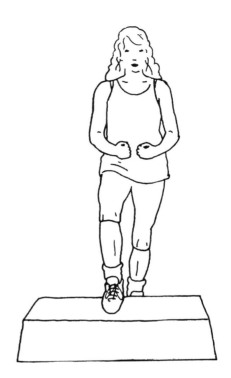

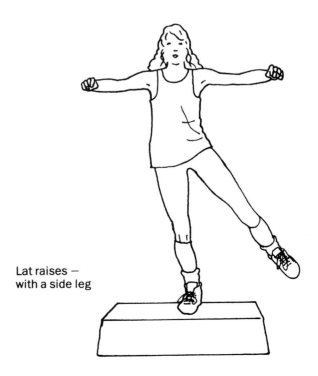

Lat raises – with a side leg

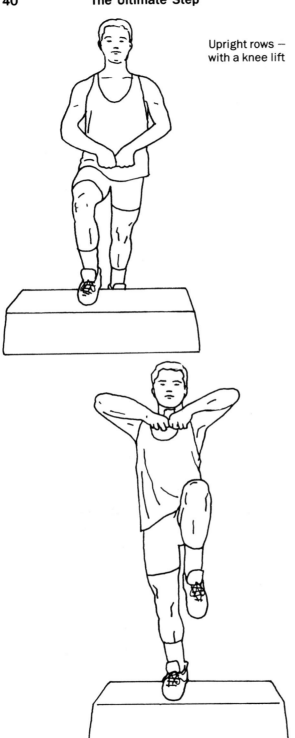

Upright rows —
with a knee lift

are holding on to a bar. Once again, pull straight upward through your elbows, not relying on your biceps, so that your hands end up at chin height – no higher. You should feel the muscles in your shoulders contract as you shrug your shoulders up and squeeze your elbows back slightly. Lower your arms slowly and with control to end the movement.

As with the lat raises, master the movement first and only then increase the pace, pulling upward to the count of one as you step up with the right, and pressing downward to the count of two as your left foot joins in, repeating this action as you step off the platform again.

The Chest

And so to the chest, where the pectorals – a kind of armour plating across your ribcage – can be worked through different combinations of *presses* – why not try a few chest presses, pushing your arms out in front of you at chest level? – and movements like *flyes* and *pec decks*.

Flyes

Begin with your arms extended out to the sides, palms facing downward, at about shoulder height so that you feel a slight stretch in your chest. Make sure that your elbows are soft, and neck, shoulders and arms relaxed – you are not working these at the moment. Slowly flex your pectoral muscles, squeezing them hard so that you draw your arms together in front of you and across your chest before releasing the contraction and pulling them back out again to the starting position. Try not to cheat and use your arm muscles during the inward squeeze, really focusing on the chest so that you begin toning it up.

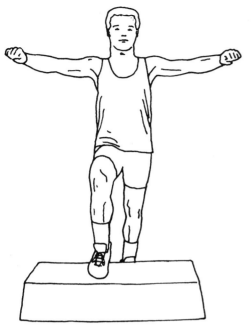

Flyes — with normal stepping

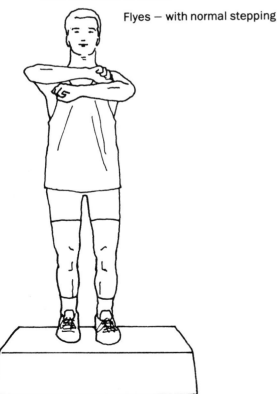

Pec Deck

Now, developing this movement one stage further, when you hold your arms out to the sides this time, bend them at the elbows so that your hands are pointing upward with your palms facing the front. When you contract your pecs, think about leading your arms inward through your elbows until they touch in the middle. Indeed, you might even give them an extra little squeeze when your arms meet, but whatever you do, remember to keep your elbows high and to extend them fully when you draw your arms apart again, so working your pecs from full stretch to total contraction. It is tempting to try to extend the outward stretch by arching the back — but as always, keep your buttocks tucked well in and body line intact.

If this is enough for you for now, go on to the cool-down section in Chapter Nine (p 77).

The First Routine

You've mastered the basic steps and got the hang of the upper-body work. It's now time to put the two together in a short routine. This will be split into two sections, each of which lasts about seven or eight minutes. Work through the first section twice only to begin with so that it becomes quite familiar and you don't need to look at the book. For reference, a skeleton version of this routine is on p 108 if you have problems remembering the sequence. Then next time, work through the second section a couple of times and, when you have practised both and can remember which step follows what and which arm movement goes with which leg exercise, join the two together into one longer workout.

If you are not used to exercising, having practised all these new steps you may well

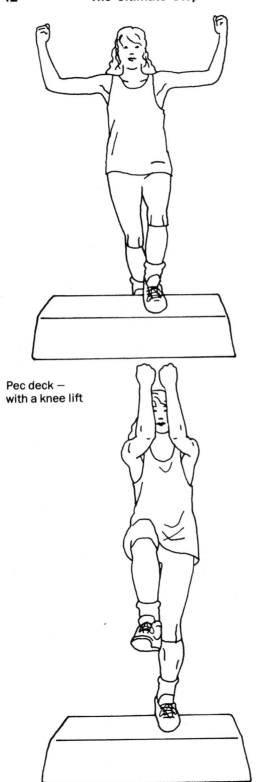

Pec deck —
with a knee lift

only be able to go through the first section once, and may not be able to manage all the different arm movements in combination with the legs. Don't worry. Put your hands on your hips and add the movements bit by bit, starting on section two when you're ready and gradually building the routine up. Then, when you can do the whole thing in one go, you can always do it twice in a row to work yourself that little bit harder. After all, fitness is about progression – *your* progression. Never overstrain yourself but always make sure that, whatever you do manage to achieve, your technique is correct and that you concentrate on the various leg and arm movements fully, working them – and never allowing *them* to work *you*!

So, make sure that you are properly warmed up and take a quick sip of water just in case your body needs it – better to be safe than sorry! Then take a deep breath and start squatting gently up and down behind your bench with your hands on your hips.

The First-timer's Routine

Work in sets of 16 for all the steps that follow – 16 on your right then 16 on your left so that your routine is balanced but no single movement practised for too long at any given time.

1. **Start stepping up and down off the bench normally, leading with your right leg, pumping your arms by your sides and watching your technique. Tap down to change to your left and continue stepping.**

2. **Tap down again and continue stepping on your right, introducing a bicep curl at half-speed. Tap down again and change legs, doing the bicep curls at normal speed now.**

3. Tap down once more and repeat this with half- and full-speed upright rows.

4. It's time to work those buttocks a little more now so tap down again and start the V-step on the right, placing your hands on your hips and concentrating on those legs. Come on! Use your full bench and really squeeze those muscles.

   Tap down once more, introducing flyes when you've got into the rhythm.

5. Change legs with a tap down once again and now introduce the wide step to work those buttocks even more. Pump your arms again, tapping down as before to change legs and maintaining the same arms.

6. Tap down and return to the simple V-step once more, still pumping the arms vigorously.

7. Tap down once more — and keep tapping, alternating the legs so that they work evenly. Try introducing the tricep kick-back at half-speed, really squeezing the back of your arms.

8. Bring your legs together in the centre of the bench and keep tapping, still working with the tricep kick-back but at full speed now or, if you're getting tired, simply pumping your arms.

9. Return to straight stepping leading with the right with a bicep curl, before tapping down and working on the left with the tricep kick-back.

10. Tap down and continue stepping normally (on the right), pumping your arms by your sides before rounding off the first half by tapping down and working on the left.

Now either return to the beginning so that you practise the sequence all over again before moving on to the next section or, if you are stopping now, go straight into the cool-down section in Chapter Nine (p 77). If you are continuing with the sequence below, make sure that you are happy with the footwork before introducing any arm movements. You can always add them next time through. Remember — you are trying to learn the routine at this stage. There is plenty of time to work your upper body later.

11. Move straight into the alternate tap up beginning on your right, pumping your arms vigorously and watching your technique carefully all the time.

12. Introduce the chest press and continue tapping up with every step.

13. Now move into the alternate knee lift, pumping your arms. When you do this section again next time, you might like to introduce a bicep curl here so that knees and forearms are raised simultaneously.

14. Change this to a leg curl, possibly with a tricep kick-back on the next time through. As with the knee lift and bicep curl above, this is a good combination because both involve a backward movement, squeezing the limb behind — so get used to it!

15. It's time for the low, controlled side leg with a comparable lateral-moving arm action — either lat raises or flyes, or, if you feel like it, your hands on your hips.

16. Return to the simple tap up, pumping your arms vigorously.

17. It's back for a final blast of knee lifts, this time with pec deck.

18. And once more to simple alternate tapping up, pumping your arms vigorously.

19. **Now start stepping normally with a chest press, leading with the right before changing legs with a knee lift.**

20. **And back to straight stepping with your hands on your hips, leading with your left before a final tap down and rounding everything off by straight stepping leading with your right, tapping down and leading with your left.**

Now march behind your bench with your hands on your hips.

Go to the cool-down section in Chapter Nine (p 77) and stretch yourself out a bit to prevent your body from getting stiff. Then, why not try a few simple strength-training exercises for added muscle tone and conditioning?

You are now an official stepper — so welcome. You've mastered the basics, can combine simple arm and leg routines and you are listening to your body for any telltale signs of discomfort. All you need to do now is have a refreshing drink, look piously at the biscuit tin — and get ready to do it all again in a couple of days' time! You may well discover that, for all their seeming simplicity, these first steps have worked you a lot harder than you thought.

chapter seven

Turning Up the Heat

A More Intensive Workout

THIS IS WHERE the fun really starts. A bench has four sides — and we're going to use them. The fairly static face-on approach is all very well for starters, but what about the main course, the bit which gets you steaming?

By now you should have mastered all the basic steps and arm movements, be able to change the leading leg without thinking about it and have perfected your technique so that it has become second nature. You're well on the road to a good level of fitness. So what now?

A Three-part Approach

The following exercises in this chapter will be divided into three sections — those which develop the work face-on to the bench, those with which you approach the bench from the side and finally, those which make use of the end of the bench — each of which concludes

with a short routine incorporating all the latest moves.

As always, listen to your body and, if at any time you feel uncomfortably winded or find a step pattern too demanding, return to pumping your arms with the simple alternate tap up until you have brought your pulse rate back down to a more appropriate level. And if you still find the going a bit tough, lower your bench a little if you can. Remember — if your body is too tired, your technique will start to deteriorate and not only will you risk injury, but all that effort will go to waste.

So keep your posture lifted, your stomach and pelvis tucked in and your upper body relaxed and balanced as you once more start marching that body to a leaner and more toned condition.

Make sure that you have warmed up thoroughly before you begin any of the sections below and that you are quite familiar with the foot patterns before adding any arms. Practise each step – or step combination – at least eight times and always work both sides equally. Remember – the better you know each movement, the easier the routines will be to follow.

STEP ONE
Working the Bench Face-on

Travelling Steps

Benchwork is not just about a static stepping up and down from behind the centre of your platform – although as you know, this in itself can be testing enough. Introduce a few travelling steps which involve working from one end of the bench to the other and your whole routine suddenly shifts up a gear, becoming that much more demanding – as well as allowing you to

all the various leg movements together into
re interesting combinations.

The Travelling Tap Up

So, after squatting up and down gently behind your bench, start stepping normally for a few counts with your hands on your hips, before introducing the alternate tap up in the centre of your bench.

Now, the next time you tap up with your right foot, shrug your left shoulder forward, turning the whole of your upper body inward towards your tapping foot. When you tap up with your left foot, the right shoulder shrugs forward. Now exaggerate the shrug so that your whole body turns when you tap up. Then, when you feel confident about this movement, start stepping up with your right foot on to the top left-hand corner of your bench and your left foot on to the top right-hand corner. You are working along the diagonal each time, stepping wide behind your bench to take you from end to end – all the time travelling with a tap up.

The Travelling Knee Lift

Increase the intensity by changing the simple tap up into a knee lift at each end of the bench. Come on – it's not enough just to get that foot a few inches off the platform. Work those thighs and lift your knees up. Keep the heel of your supporting foot well pressed down and stand tall, lifting out of your hips with strong abdominal muscles, but making sure that your supporting knee is never locked out.

Punch it Out

The travelling knee lift is a strong movement – so when you've got into the rhythm of it, start punching your arms out alternately in front of you at chest height so that your upper body begins to work too.

Climb the Rope

Continue travelling from end to end along your bench but this time start 'climbing the rope', a vigorous arm movement which will really get that blood moving.

Imagine that there is a rope in front of you and pull down on it from above head height with alternate arms so that they pass each other in a scissor-type movement. Resist the action both up and down and really get that body moving.

The Travelling Leg Curl

Now change the knee lift into a leg curl at each end of the bench, squeezing the hamstrings hard every time and maybe introducing the tricep kick-back after a few steps as you practised in the previous chapter. Alternatively, with both arms raised above your head, pull down strongly in a wide arc – a *lateral pull-down* – so that your hands finish up at waist height out to the sides

Climbing the rope —
with a travelling knee lift

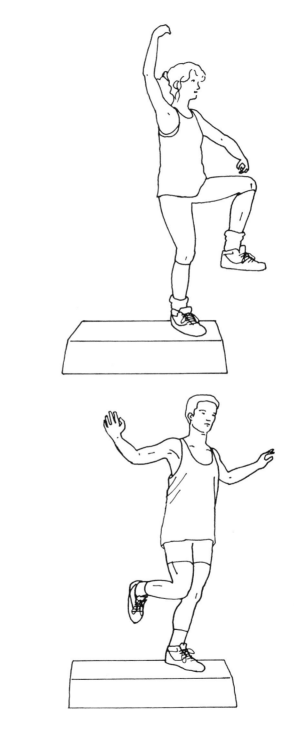

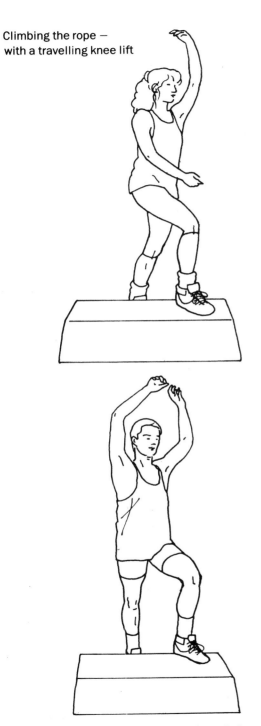

The travelling leg curl — with a lateral pull-down

with your elbows slightly bent and palms facing the front before returning them to their starting position. If you are working in front of a mirror, check your body position regularly to make sure that you are not arching your back and that your neck stays relaxed.

The Travelling Side Leg

And when you're happy that your technique is perfect, change this once more into the low, controlled side leg — that squeezing action with the foot flexed and facing the front — remembering to keep your hips square and buttocks tight. As before, introduce some flyes with this leg movement to work your chest a little more. Or, to widen your repertoire of arm movements, try a few bicep curls with your arms at shoulder height out to the sides, palms facing the ceiling. As with normal arm curls, keep the biceps flexed the whole time by never fully extending the elbow joints, and really squeeze the movement both in and out so you make those muscles work.

The Buttock Basher

Most of the footwork you have learned so far involves the forward lifting action of the leg using the so-called 'hip flexors'. To balance this out, therefore, try this exercise which uses the 'hip extensors' by lifting your leg out behind you.

Very similar to the side leg in that it is a small, pressing action relying on the amount you squeeze your buttocks rather than how high you raise your foot, the buttock basher really gives those gluteal muscles a going over.

When you step up on to the bench, flex the trailing foot and raise it a couple of inches — no more — behind you, supporting yourself by squeezing your abdominal muscles and extending both arms in front of you for balance.

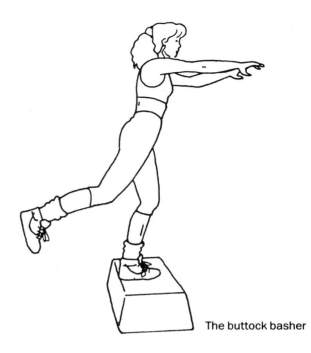

The buttock basher

It is a small movement, not a wide swing, and you should practise it a few times on each side to perfect your technique.

Then start travelling from end to end along the bench, and introduce it as with all the other movements.

The Shuffle

This is a simple variation on the travelling knee lift which brings the end of the bench into use for the first time, by simply adding a tap down and knee lift at each end.

So begin with the travelling knee lift once again, swinging from side to side four times until you end up with your left knee raised at the left-hand side of the bench. This time, instead of simply stepping back off behind you once again, square your body to face the front and step out to the side and off the end with your left foot. Tap down with your right and step up with it into another knee lift with your left leg.

Then continue as for the straight travelling knee lift – stepping down with the left behind you, along with the right and up with the left at the other end of the bench, this time raising your right knee up to waist height. Again, step off the end of the platform with that leg, tapping down and stepping up again with the left, and bringing the right straight back up into a knee lift once more as you return to your starting position.

As always, practise the whole pattern at least eight times, introducing upper body movements as soon as you feel fit. What about maintaining a chest press throughout, but adding a shoulder press every time you do a knee lift, so mirroring the upward movement in both arms and legs?

The shoulder press – with a knee lift

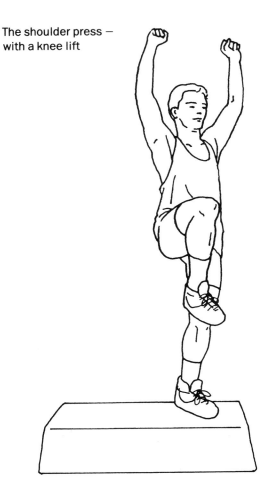

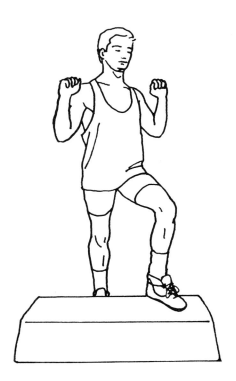

Shoulder Press

Bring both hands up to shoulder height about twice shoulder width apart with your elbows pointing straight down to the floor and knuckles to the ceiling. Without arching your back, and making sure that your stomach and buttocks are well tucked in, press your hands vertically upward to the ceiling, squeezing your shoulder blades together a fraction and resisting the movement as much as you can. Then, just before your elbows lock out, draw your arms back down again, keeping your shoulder blades pressed together. Practise this as a four-count movement until you are confident about it and then do it in two counts when you add it to the shuffle, drawing both arms up as you step up into the knee lift and down as you descend.

Repeaters

The main way to increase the intensity of a movement, however, is to repeat it on the same leg, one time after another, so that the given muscles are worked through that particular range of motion three or five times in succession – no more than that.

Go back to the travelling knee lift for a couple more steps but, the next time you go to step up with your right, plant it even more firmly than normal, really pushing down through your heel and not bouncing up on to your toes with the momentum, and do three knee lifts in a row on your left. Remember to keep your chest well lifted, your pelvis tilted in and the knee of your supporting leg soft – and don't cheat by only raising your left knee halfway. Take it all the way up every time so that your left thigh is really made to work, and make sure that you land carefully on the floor with your left foot each time, the ball of the foot melting downward into the heel and onward into a gentle knee bend, so cushioning the impact on your joints, whilst giving yourself a sufficient springboard to power yourself up into the next knee lift.

Then step down and across to the right-hand end of the bench to repeat the movement with the right knee.

Practise each side alternately for a few minutes – and add upright rows when you feel confident enough. Then, when you've got it all sussed, vary this with reps (repeaters) of three leg curls – punching out alternately with right and left arms at chest height – and reps of three side legs with lat raises, concentrating on your technique

the whole time and making sure that you don't arch your back.

You will immediately notice the increase in intensity that this simple alteration to the basic step brings – so make the most of it and really work those legs. When it comes to the routine proper, you'll be doing reps of five anyway – the upper limit that you can safely do because of the potential strain that any movement such as this can put on your knees.

Adductor Touch

Another variation that you might like to think about is a development of the knee lift. By

The adductor touch

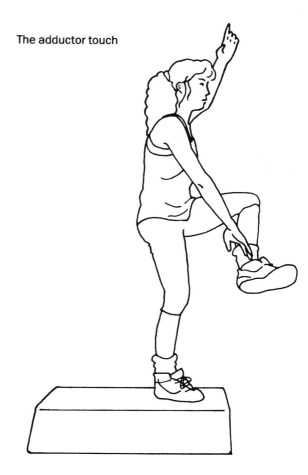

modifying it so that you draw your right leg across your body slightly and touch your right foot with both hands in front of you and vice versa, you focus attention on to your adductors – your inner thighs – and so attack your legs from a different angle. Now, when you have got the feel of the movement, test your co-ordination a little more by raising the arm on the working side so that only your right hand touches your left foot and vice versa. A teasing little variation!

Practise a couple more reps of three with this variation, but don't overdo it if you're getting tired.

Turn Step

One of my favourites, this is a particularly useful step to master because it uses the full length of the bench – so maintaining the high aerobic workout – and also allows you to link movements which work the bench face-on with those which work the bench side-on. However, if you have weak knees, be very careful. The pivoting action of this movement may put them under stress.

Pump your arms and continue stepping as normal, introducing the V-step after a few moments and then tapping down on each side alternately. Gradually start to swing your body from side to side, easing over to your left when you tap down with your left, to your right when you tap down with your right so that eventually you swing right round from end to end on your bench, turning your body to face the right wall at the left-hand end and the left wall at the right-hand end.

Practise this as usual, using the full length of the bench, and after a few times introduce lat raises, to balance the sideways movement along the top of the bench.

Turn Step – With a Lunge

To work yourself even harder, lunge your foot back instead of simply tapping it down at each end of the bench. Come on – put a bit of effort into it! Bend that supporting leg and work those buttocks – but be careful not to force your heel down to the ground on your extended leg.

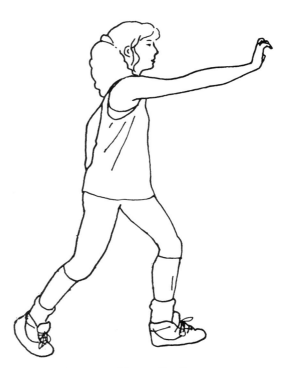

The basic lunge position on the floor

Press and Punch

And now add reps of three lunges on each side, punching out the arm on the working side of the body at chest height in front of you to increase the aerobic demand even more. And when you step up and along the bench as normal, introduce a shoulder press to spice things up here too. Bend those knees and don't cheat on the lunges. Keep your weight centred well over the supporting leg and remember – the harder you work, the more calories you burn up!

The Face-On Routine

Making good use of those energy reserves, it's time to work body and brain together now in a workout which will test both a little more. Of course, if you want to hang up your trainers at this point and pick this all up again in a couple of days' time – fine. You can always squeeze those abdominals a bit in Chapter Ten – or even wind up totally with your full cool-down if you want. If not, take a drink now, mop your brow and start working through the following pages. The routine should take about seven or eight minutes – vigorous minutes – so if you find the going a bit tough, place your hands on your hips again or lower the height of your bench a little if you can. Concentrate on your technique throughout, and always keep your stomach and buttocks tucked in. As before, use the Appendices for reference if you find the sequence difficult to remember.

Make sure that you are fully warmed up before attempting this workout, and that you have mobilized and stretched out both arms and legs properly.

1. Squat gently up and down in front of your bench with your hands on your hips for four beats and then start stepping normally, leading with your right leg and introducing a bicep curl. Keep your elbows in close to your sides and squeeze the muscles hard with every contraction. Tap down and begin again on the left, changing the arms to tricep kick-backs once the left leg is leading.
   Repeat 16 times on each side

2. Pump your arms and introduce the alternate tap up starting on the right as before, moving into alternate knee lifts after eight steps. Do a chest press as you step up, and lower your arms to touch the front of your thighs as you step back off again. Step up – arms out. Step down – arms down.
   Repeat 16 times

3. Now start swinging from side to side into the travelling knee lift, changing your arms into a shoulder press when you've found your rhythm. Remember – you are working on the diagonal so that when your right leg leads, you travel across to the left-hand side of the bench and vice versa.
   Repeat 8 times

4. This time increase the intensity into sets of three knee lifts as you travel from side to side, pulling your arms down from above your head to waist height as practised with the lateral pull-down.
   Repeat 4 times – two reps of three on each side

5. Now work your way through all the different leg movements you know, with reps of three adductor touches, both hands touching your raised foot – or with one hand raised if you feel like it – three leg curls with a tricep kick-back, three side legs with lat raises and three buttock bashers pumping your arms. This'll be tough, so concentrate on pressing your heel down firmly on to the bench throughout.
   Repeat each rep of three 4 times – twice on each leg

6. Return to the travelling tap up to ease off a bit, still pumping your arms.
   Repeat 8 times

7. As you travel over to your left once more, introduce the shuffle. Step off the end of your bench with your left after the knee lift,

tapping down with your right before stepping up on to it again into a knee lift on the left as you travel back the other side. Simply pump your arms to begin with and then introduce the chest press/shoulder press combination you practised earlier.

Repeat 8 times

8. Forget the added tap down and knee lift and go back to the straight travelling knee lift again for four, before returning to the centre once more to stay facing the front with the simple alternate tap up, pumping your arms.

Repeat 8 times

9. Start stepping normally, leading with your right leg, and pump your arms before tapping down.

Repeat 8 times on each side

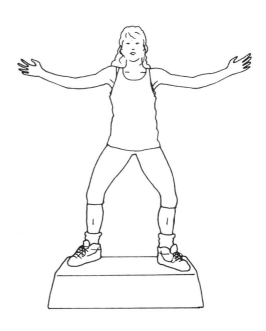

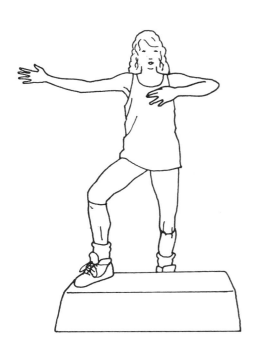

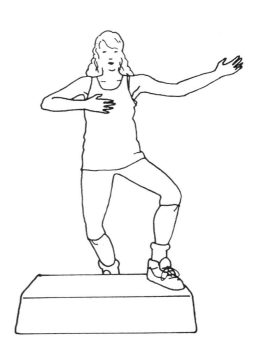

The V-step — with arms following legs

10. Now introduce the wide V-step, allowing your arms to follow your legs — that is, as you step out wide to the right, you lift your right arm out to shoulder height at your side and hold it there as you raise your left arm out as your left foot steps up, lowering them first right then left as you step back down again. Tap down to change the leading leg.

   Repeat 8 times on each side

11. Tap down again with your right and move into alternate V-step. Double the arms so that both are extended out to your sides at shoulder height and drawn back in again with every step.

   Repeat 16 times

12. Pump your arms and change this into a turn step so that you gradually turn your whole body to face the right-hand wall as you step off with the right, tapping down at the left-hand end of your bench. Continue with the turn step as normal over to the left.

   It's a tricky changeover the first time round, but you'll get it right next time.

   Introduce a chest press if you can, pushing your arms out in front of you every time you step along the top of the board and with every tap down.

   Repeat 16 times

13. As you go to tap down with your left this time, extend it out to a lunge behind you, introducing the press-and-punch arm sequence that you practised before.

   Repeat 8 times

14. Add reps of three lunges, with the same press-and-punch arms.

   Repeat 4 times

15. Pump your arms and return to the normal turn step for seven more steps. Then stay off your bench, pulsing gently up and down with your hands on your hips at the left-hand end of your bench.

As always, either return to the beginning for practice, or wind yourself down a bit (Chapter Nine, p 77) before going on to the strength-training work.

STEP TWO
Working the Bench Side-on

Moving from side to side across the bench adds a variety of new steps to your repertoire, steps which always seem more exhausting but help to shape up your outer and inner thighs more. These are my favourite movements because the choreography is far less static, using all four sides of the bench.

Stand behind the centre of your bench and turn to your right so that your left side is closest to the platform. Until you have a feel for the type of movements involved, practise everything at half-speed, concentrating on your technique all the way. Then, as before, repeat each new movement at least eight times on each side so that you really have got the hang of it.

Traversing

This step basically crosses over the bench and back again, working both legs evenly. To begin it, stand with your hands on your hips and, as always, squat gently up and down in time to the music.

On the count of four, step up to your left with your left foot, planting it slightly in front of you on the bench so that your knee is more or less above your ankle. Make sure that the heel is firmly placed and bring the right foot up beside it. Transfer your full weight on to this side —

making sure you don't lock your knees out – and continue the movement over the top, stepping gently off the bench a fraction behind you on to the ball of your left foot, lowering yourself on to the heel and tapping down with your right.

Bring your right foot straight back up on to the bench again and repeat the action in the other direction so that you end up in your starting position.

Try to keep your hips square throughout and don't lean excessively forward when you step up but maintain a good body line, with your upper body relaxed and neck and spine long. And when you are sure about your technique, start working the step at normal speed, introducing a bicep curl or chest press when you're ready. After just a few short minutes of practice, you'll notice the different demands that traversing makes of your legs.

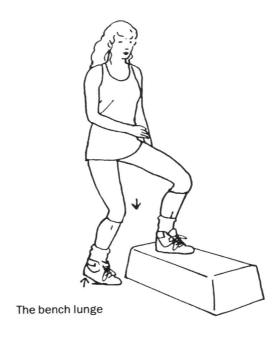

The bench lunge

The Bench Lunge

This movement is surprisingly demanding, for all its apparent simplicity. So stand on top of your bench facing down it lengthways to your right, and squat gently up and down with your hands on your hips.

From this relaxed position, turn slightly to your left and lunge down on the diagonal to the right-hand side of the bench with your right foot on the count of one, so that your right leg is extended behind you, melting down into the ball of your foot so that both legs are bent. Hold it there for the count of one – keeping your weight well over your supporting leg but without bending forward from the waist – and then return to your starting position for two more counts before repeating the action on your left.

Continue on alternate sides until you feel confident about the action and only then carry on in double time, taking one count for every stage of the movement. At this speed you may not be able to roll down on to your heel so, if it feels more comfortable, keep the heel of your lunging foot off the floor.

Remember – always bend your supporting leg, with your outstretched foot fairly close into your bench so that you don't overstress the Achilles tendon running down from your calf to your ankle.

After just a few short lunges like this, the front of your thighs and your buttocks will really begin to feel the workload. And if they don't, it's not because you're super-fit – far from it. It just means that you're cutting corners. So bend those knees and really work. No feeble tap downs! You're only cheating yourself if you take it easy. If you do have weak knees, though, keep a careful watch-out for even the slightest hint of discomfort and stop immediately if you feel you should.

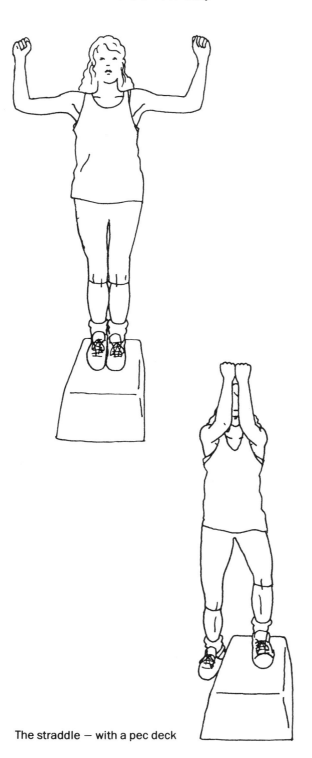

Lunging Reps

This time, instead of simply doing one lunge on each side of the bench, repeat the action four times before changing over so that you increase the intensity of the movement.

The Straddle

While the lunge is primarily a one-legged move-ment, the straddle brings both legs into play. From your squatting position looking length-ways down the bench, step down to the right slightly behind you with your right foot, landing carefully with the ball of the foot first followed by the heel, and bending your knees a touch to cushion the impact. With your foot firmly planted, step down to the left-hand side of the bench with your left foot parallel to your right so that the bench is between your legs. Keep

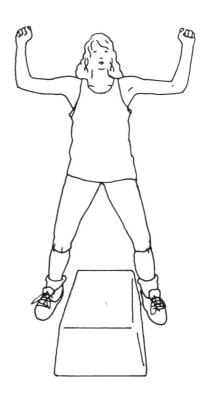

The straddle — with a pec deck

your knees soft, stomach pulled in and don't arch your back.

Step up again with your right foot slightly in front of you again so that your knee is directly over your ankle, not forward over your toes which would make it tempting to take your heel off the bench. Bring your left foot up too so that you are back to your starting position, once more bringing your feet parallel to each other, with your knees soft and heels pressed down into the platform. Practise the movement a few times, tap the top of the bench and repeat it leading with your left leg this time.

The pec deck is a good arm exercise to try with this one – but don't arch your back when you step down.

Alternate Straddle Step

As with straight stepping, the simple straddle only really works one leg at a time, so the more usual way to use it during routines is to tap up every time the trailing foot approaches the bench so that you change the leading leg.

Start squatting gently on top of your bench once more and introduce the straddle step, leading with your right leg. This time, as your left leg comes up, simply tap on top of the bench with it and step straight back down to the floor again. Step down on the right-hand side with your right foot as well, bringing the left foot back up on to the bench as usual. Then, as before, simply tap up with the right, continuing to change the leading leg at the end of each straddle so that both legs work evenly.

Once you are confident about the movement, make your upper body work a little more by adding flyes to the equation, squeezing the chest every time your trailing leg reaches the floor and the bench.

The Squatting Straddle

This movement is a little tricky to get right, but the benefits for your thighs and buttocks are tremendous so it is worth taking a bit of time over it.

Go back to pumping your arms and straddling with alternate legs. Then, the next time you go to straddle down, step out wide on each side into a gentle squat before continuing with the straddle movement as practised. Your body position is crucial here so you should definitely work it through in slow motion, watching your profile in the mirror as you go.

When you move into the squat, your feet should be pointing slightly outward and knees travelling directly over them. All your weight should be pushed down through your heels, your body in a natural upright position with your neck and spine in line. All the work should be on your thighs and buttocks and, as long as your body position is correct, you should feel no pressure on either your knees or your lower back. If you do – modify your alignment accordingly. And if you feel any discomfort at all during this movement, stop immediately and return to the straight straddle.

However, if you have got it right, carry on working the movement at full speed. You will feel a build-up of tension in your thighs fairly quickly, so don't overdo things at this stage. Remember – you are only practising these exercises at the moment so that you perfect your technique. You are not doing a full-blown workout.

Alternate Straddle Step – With a Knee Lift

As with the simple alternate tap up that you learnt in the previous chapter, the alternate straddle step can be developed using knee lifts, leg curls and side legs. All you have to do is

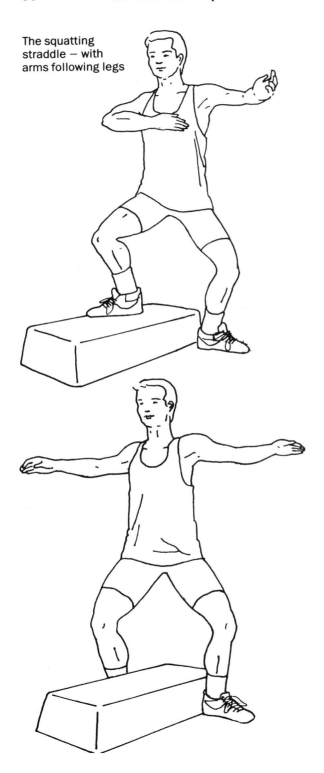

The squatting straddle — with arms following legs

substitute one of those movements for every tap up so that you are still changing the leading leg but are working your body that little bit harder. Keep your feet firmly planted, hips square and don't arch your back, and try a few variations until you feel confident about every move.

Alternate Straddle Step — With Reps

Once you've mastered this you can always add reps of three and five on each side to work yourself even harder still.

To begin with, work with the side leg, doing two sets of three — one on each side of the bench — before pushing your knee out to the side and introducing the adductor touch so that you work your inner thighs a bit more. Try a couple of sets of this as well and then alternate between the two, working the inner and outer thigh muscles alternately to tone up the whole area.

Then swap these for alternating sets of three knee lifts and three leg curls, tightening up the front and back of your thighs this time. Pump your arms vigorously throughout.

The Straddling Sequence

We are now going to join the traverse and the straddle steps together in a great little combination which should definitely make you step up and think! So practise it thoroughly. It'll make your life a lot easier when it comes to the routines ahead.

a. **Return to the straight traverse for four more steps, leading with your left.**

b. **Add a straddle**
Begin the traverse as normal but, when both feet are on top of your bench, straddle down and up with your lead-

ing leg, and then continue with the traverse as before.

Tap down and repeat the whole movement on the other side, practising this pattern eight times — or more, if you find it difficult. Lower the height of your bench if you are finding the going a bit tough but never let your technique suffer. Keep your heels pressed well down and land gently on each side, rolling through from the ball to the heel to cushion your joints.

c. Introduce a squat
    If you mastered this movement earlier, turn the straddle into a squat — watching your body position carefully all the time! Keep your legs wide and push down through your heels with your weight well centred.

d. Add a knee lift
    When you are confident about the sequence so far, it's time to raise the intensity by adding a knee lift at the start of each traverse. So, the next time you tap down with your left, step up with it again as normal but do a knee lift with your right, before tapping down with your left once more and starting the traverse—straddle/squat pattern as before. Again, as you tap down with your right on the other side, add a knee lift on the left before tapping down once more and continuing with the sequence, practising this at least 16 times.

It takes a bit of getting used to, but this is a terrific combination to master because it really does work all the major muscle groups in the lower body. Don't overdo it, though,

and gradually wind down again, taking away first the knee lifts for four more traverses, then the squats (if you are including them) and finally the straddle so that you are simply crossing over the bench and back again for a final four steps.

The Side-on Routine

It's time to put all these new moves together in a fairly intense routine, lasting about seven or eight minutes, which focuses on working the bench from the side. All the steps will be familiar to you, as well as some of the patterns, so concentrate fully on your technique at all stages and turn straight to Appendix 2 (pp109–10) if you can't remember the sequence of steps from start to finish. Take a quick sip of water so that you are in no danger of dehydrating — you've been working pretty hard over the last few minutes — and as always, bring your arms down on to your hips as soon as you feel the workout becoming too intense.

Make sure that you have warmed up fully before attempting this workout and that you have stretched out your arms and legs properly.

1. Stand facing the right behind your bench and, after squatting gently up and down a few times with your hands on your hips, start traversing the bench, pumping your arms vigorously.

    Repeat 16 times

2. Add a knee lift each side before tapping down and traversing the bench as usual. Climb the rope when you have got into your rhythm.

    Repeat 16 times

3. Now add reps of five knee lifts on each side of the bench, tapping down and traversing as

before in between. Introduce the pec deck to start working the chest a bit more – but keep those elbows high!

Repeat 4 times – twice on each side

4. Go back to single knee lifts with a traverse and add a straddle in the middle as you practised with the straddle sequence. Introduce the chest press.

Repeat 8 times

5. Now incorporate a squat if you can, taking great care with your technique – wide stance, knees over your feet, strong back, weight pressed down through the heels. This time do a shoulder press every time you go down, continuing with the chest press for all other leg movements. If you can't manage this, continue with the simple straddle.

Repeat 8 times

6. Replace the squat with a straddle for four more steps and then move into a continuous straddle step leading with your left leg. Tap up and repeat on the other side, climbing the rope with your arms and placing your feet carefully each time.

Repeat 8 times on each side

7. Then, when both feet are on top of the bench once more, start the alternate lunge down on your left, pressing the arm of your working side out in front of you at chest height.

Repeat 8 times

8. Move straight into reps of four lunges on each side, starting on your left. This time push upward above your head with your working arm, lifting out of your abdomen so that you get a good stretch down each side in turn.

Repeat 4 times on each side

9. Return to single lunges, punching out with your arm at chest height on the working side once again.

Repeat 8 times

10. The next time you bring your right foot back up on to the bench again, straddle down, leading with the left, introducing lat raises. Tap up and repeat on the right this time, maintaining the same arms.

Repeat 8 times on each side

11. Tap up – and keep tapping, introducing alternate straddle steps on your left with upright rows.

Repeat 16 times

12. Now introduce squats with a shoulder press if you can. Alternatively, try the straddle step with a knee lift, introducing a bicep curl.

Repeat 8 times

13. Return to alternate straddle step, pumping the arms.

Repeat 16 times

14. For a final blast, this time lunge down to your left and up, then down to your right and up, and only then straddle down fully to your left. Tap up with your right, and then lunge down to your right and up, then your left and up, straddling down to your right and continuing to work this pattern on each side alternately.

Repeat 8 times

15. On the last time you lunge down on your right, step down fully on this side, tap down with your left and start traversing with your left foot. This time work your upper body with a tricep kick-back before ending up squatting gently by your bench with your hands on your hips.

Repeat 8 times

So it's back to the start again for practice, or a couple of minutes' winding down (see Chapter Nine) before a quick jaunt through the abdominal work and strength-training section, or off for a full cool-down and stretch-out in time for a long refreshing drink and invigorating shower. Any combination of these sounds good to me.

STEP THREE
Working the Bench End-on

With your T-shirt nicely damp and your adrenalin really buzzing, this final group of steps works the bench facing down it lengthways. So start stepping normally with your right leg, pumping those arms for all they're worth.

T-Step

You'll really enjoy this movement which combines the straight step with the straddle that you learnt earlier.

Begin stepping normally, leading with your right leg. Then, halfway through the eighth step when both feet are on top of your bench, start straddling down, again leading with the right. After eight of these, step backward off your bench and start stepping normally once again, this time just for four. Halfway through the fourth step, start straddling down once more, stepping off backward after the fourth, and repeating this combination in doubles, then finally singles so that you step up, straddle down, step back up again and step off – tracing a T-shape with your feet.

Repeat it a few times and then tap down with your left, to start from the beginning again leading with the opposite leg.

Alternate T-Step

You've probably guessed already but, as with all the other exercises, the T-step can be developed to work both legs equally by tapping down *every* time you step back off the end of your bench, so changing the leading leg. Try it for a while.

Alternate T-step — With a Knee Lift

A good development of the T-step is to add any one of the different leg movements that you are now familiar with – be it a knee lift, leg curl, side leg or buttock basher – in a combination which you'll probably need to build up gradually, since it can be a little confusing first time through.

Start the alternate tap down, leading into the alternate T-step as before. This time, though, step up with your right, *tap up* with your left and step straight down with your left into your straddle. Continue normally with the straddle until you lift your right foot up on the bench once more and again *tap it up* before stepping back off with it. Tap down with your left and step up with it again, repeating the whole thing on the other side – that is, tapping up every time your trailing foot approaches the bench. A bit of practice is probably called for here!

Now, with everything going in the right place at the right time, simply substitute one of your leg movements – try the side leg since it follows the lateral movement of the straddle step – squeezing the left leg outward on the count of two as you step up on to the bench with your right and stepping straight off the bench again on that side into a straddle without letting your left foot touch the bench. Similarly, as you step up again with your left foot at the end of the straddle, move directly into a side leg on your right this time, before completing the T-shape with the backward step off the bench and tapping down. At no point are there two feet on the bench together.

And when you've got that little lot sussed, complement this small controlled action with a lateral arm movement – like the shoulder-height bicep curl or, indeed, flyes or lat raises. Alternatively, if you try it with the knee lift, what about combining it with the pec deck, but adding a small twist to the movement. Every time you draw your knee up towards your waist, turn your entire torso gently to that side so that you touch your knee with the opposite elbow. Straddle down working the chest muscles as normal and again, touch your knee with the opposite elbow as you do the knee lift on the other side. It will begin working the oblique muscles down each side of your torso and so help to tighten up your waist. Squeeze the muscles as you turn – but never jerk the upper body round – and keep your hips square at all times. It is a smooth, controlled movement designed to trim back that midriff – not put you in traction for six months!

The End-on Routine

With a glass of water or cyclist's water-bottle in hand, it's time to think about the final routine in this chapter, working the bench from all angles and all directions and really making that body move. If you've done the preceding workouts, you may well be getting a bit tired – this last routine will last almost ten minutes – so lower your bench a little if necessary and concentrate extra hard on squeezing those muscles. Come on – don't cheat yourself at the last moment. Bend those knees and really burn off those calories. And if your memory is starting to go, don't forget Appendix 2 for the routines in brief.

Make sure that you are properly warmed up before starting this routine and take a quick drink of water.

1. Stand facing the right-hand wall behind your bench and squat gently up and down for a few beats before beginning to traverse over and back across your bench, pumping your arms vigorously. Introduce a chest press once you have found your rhythm.
Repeat 8 times

2. The next time both feet are on top of the bench, start straddling down, leading with your left. Climb that rope! Tap up and lead with the right, still working those arms in a strong, controlled movement. Move carefully towards the back end of your bench.
Repeat 8 times on each side

3. Step backward off the end with your left then right and step straight back up again leading with the left, bringing in the T-step and pumping your arms. Add a pec deck if you feel like it, squeezing those elbows together at shoulder height. Tap down and repeat on the right.
Repeat 8 times on each side

4. Tap down again and move straight into alternate T-step with flyes, tapping down every time you step off backward and landing gently with each foot as you straddle down.
Repeat 16 times

5. Now introduce a side leg every time you step up on to the bench as you practised above, before straddling straight down with that leg as normal. This time, however, add a low controlled buttock basher as you step up and off behind you. Tap down and repeat this on the other side – side leg before the straddle, and buttock basher before the step back – introducing lat raises when you've got into the rhythm of it. If your arms are getting tired, pump them at your sides, but concentrate hard on keeping those abdominal

muscles strong and that chest lifted all the time to ensure that your posture is good.
Repeat 16 times

6. Return to the normal alternate T-step, alternating between two pec decks and two flyes with your arms.
Repeat 16 times

7. Straddle down for the last time with your right leg and keep straddling. Tap up and continue on the left. Bicep curls or tricep kick-backs will be fine throughout.
Repeat 8 times on each side

8. Tap up once more, and very carefully lunge back with your right leg, bringing it back up on to the bench and then lunging down with your left, alternating your lunges and punching out each arm at chest height on the working side. Concentrate hard on good body alignment.
Repeat 16 times

9. Step off carefully to your right and start traversing once more, leading with your left and pumping your arms.
Repeat 8 times

It's time to begin the straddling sequence.

10. Add a knee lift on each side, tapping down and continuing the traverse as before, changing the arms to a chest press.
Repeat 8 times

11. Add a straddle in the middle of the traverse as well, changing the arms to a shoulder press. Squat down instead if you feel like it.
Repeat 8 times

12. Remove the straddle/squat for four more traverses so that you are traversing with a knee lift only, and then remove the knee

lift as well so that you are just crossing the bench back and forth while pumping your arms.
Repeat 8 times

13. Next time you tap down on the right-hand side of the bench, turn your whole body to face the front and start stepping normally, leading with your left leg. Tap down and change sides.
Repeat 8 times on each side

14. Tap down again and start the alternate V-step, your arms following your legs as before.
Repeat 16 times

15. And return to the centre with straight alternate stepping for 16, before staying off your bench and squatting gently up and down with your hands on your hips.

Too hot and sweaty even to consider any more exercise today? Cool down, stretch out properly and try it all again in a couple of days' time.

The total masochists among you will already have noticed that the three routines in this section can be joined together into one long routine lasting about 25 minutes. It'll take a bit of practice to remember it all, of course – and the notes at the end of this book will help jog your memory – but that's not really the point. *The Ultimate Step* is not about rigid formulae and studious repetition – far from it. The routines above used only a tiny amount of the arm and leg movements that you have learned, and these can be combined in a variety of ways, especially when it comes to creative upper-body work. Add a smattering of repeaters and the intensity increases instantly, simplify the moves and you can focus more specifically on certain muscle groups and begin developing the strength-training aspect of stepping.

But that's for the next chapter. Now's the time to go over a few of the moves again and maybe reread the dos and don'ts (pp 15–20) once more, having experienced the exercises and understood their significance a little more fully. Your control and technique will need to be at their best to benefit as much as possible from what's to come.

chapter eight

The Crunch

Steady Steps to Shape and Tone

THIS IS AN intense group of exercises designed to pinpoint and work specific groups of muscles with a view to tone and body shape. The cardiorespiratory demands may be slightly less, but this does not mean that these simple movements should be taken lightly. And the amount you move each muscle may be small, but so will the number of repetitions you can probably do. For when you've given your heart and lungs a good run for their money, it's time to start thinking a bit more about strength and conditioning.

Resist the movements all the way so that it feels as if you are working in double-slow motion, finding the muscle fibres and feeling them move. And if you can only manage a few reps to begin with – great. It means that you are doing the exercises properly and that you will achieve the results you want all the more quickly.

Tap Up-Tap Down

This step is a simple development of the basic up-up-down-down pattern at the heart of every benchwork routine – but you'll notice the difference immediately.

Begin stepping normally, pumping your arms and leading with your right leg. On the count of four, tap up with your left foot as if you are about to change the leading leg, stepping back off as usual, only this time don't transfer your weight on to your right leg as you would do normally, but simply tap down with your right leg too, bringing it straight back up on to the bench again. Tap up with the left again and down with the right so that you are focusing all the work on your right thigh. For this exercise only, keep both knees well bent to intensify the demand, keep pumping your arms and feel those muscles move.

To change the leading leg, don't tap down

with your right foot but actually step on to it, leaving your left foot free to step up and begin working on the other side.

Knee Lift-Tap Down

Increase the intensity now by replacing the tap up with a knee lift every time you step up. So go back to leading with your right foot and, on the count of four, change the tap up on your left foot into a knee lift, stepping straight back off again as usual before the tap down on the right leg. Keep your right heel pushed down into the bench, knees bent, pelvis tucked in and upper body relaxed.

Add a Lunge

Then, after about eight reps, lunge back your right foot instead of simply tapping down and really work those legs. Come on – feel those thigh muscles contract and those buttocks work. There are no half-measures for this set of movements.

You should begin to feel this fairly quickly, so step down once more with your left to change legs and start working on that left thigh now.

Tap Up-Tap Down – From the Side

Both the simple tap up-tap down and the knee lift-tap down can be done side-on to the bench to work the outer thigh and buttocks more intensely.

Stand at the left-hand end of your bench, facing right, so that your left foot is nearest to your platform. After squatting up and down to the music for four beats, step up to the side with your left foot – making sure that your heel is firmly planted and your foot is placed slightly in front of you on the bench so that your knee is above your heel – and tap up with your right

in front of you before stepping down with your right once more and tapping behind you with your left.

To change the leading leg, this time do a turn step on top of the bench leading with your left foot so that you end up facing the opposite direction, and begin stepping up side-on with your right. This time it'll obviously be your left foot tapping the bench in front of you and stepping straight off again to release your right foot for the tap behind you.

Add a Lunge and a Leg Curl

Change the leading leg again with another turn step and add the lunge and a leg curl this time, to begin working the hamstrings. You should really be feeling the front of your thighs and buttocks by now, so hang in there for a couple more reps before doing a turn step once more and switching the pressure on to your right.

The Crusher

If you found the last exercise difficult, wait until you try this one because it's an absolute killer. It is based on the same idea of pinpointing the thighs and buttocks – but the intensity of this version is such that even the most seasoned of steppers have lost it halfway and returned to the simple tap up-tap down.

So, take a deep breath and move to the left-hand end of your bench, facing it; step up and down with your right leg, pumping those arms vigorously. On the count of four, tap up-tap down, leading with your right. This time bring your left leg straight out to the side in a small controlled movement as you step up, keeping your foot low and pointing to the front, the knee of the supporting leg soft, hips square and stomach and pelvis tucked in. Don't take

The crusher

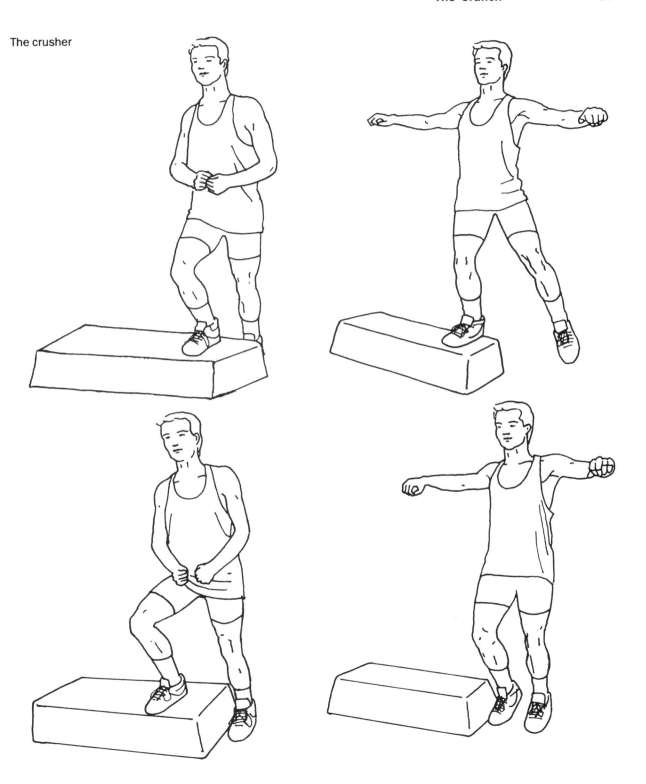

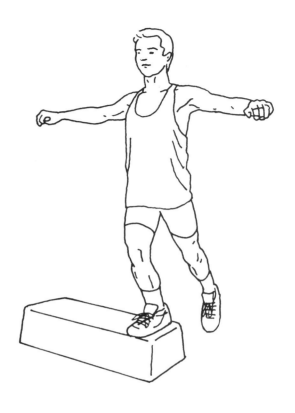

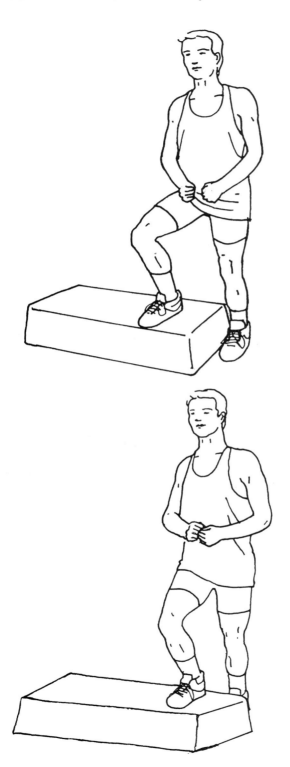

the easy option of swinging your leg out wildly to the side. Squeeze those buttocks as you go.

Now step off the end of the bench with your left leg and tap down with your right, before stepping up again with your right as usual. This time, however, draw your left leg behind you into the buttock basher, being careful not to arch your back but squeezing your left buttock hard as you do so, resisting this small action all the way. Keep your foot low again, hips square and upper body lifted, and follow the movement of your foot, stepping off the bench behind you and tapping down once more with your right foot.

Repeat this whole movement eight times to give that right thigh and left buttock a thorough work-over.

That's the easy part. Let's shift into a slightly higher gear now and bring in reps of three every time you step up on the right — that is, three reps with the leg out to the side and three reps with the leg out to the back.

A further four sets of three reps to the side and three to the back should be sufficient — but if you find the going a bit tough, return to the singles as before. There is a danger of twisting the lower back if you get too tired, so again, suck in those stomach muscles to give you a good strong foundation to the movement, keep that chest lifted, maintain a natural full-body lean — and only take the exercise as far as you can.

For the total masochists among you, though, bring the exercise to a climax with one set of five straight-leg reps. This will be tough — so don't try it unless you feel that your body can take it.

Then finish the whole thing off with two more sets of three straight-leg reps before winding it down with four more singles and eight more straight steps leading with the left — shuffling you over to the right-hand side of the bench.

Yes — it's time to repeat the whole thing on the other side. So take a deep breath, tap down with your left foot and begin the simple tap up-tap down on this side, before bringing in the crusher to focus on the front of your left thigh and right buttock. Come on, go for it! Feel the muscles and make them work.

The Slow Half-Step Squat

We are going to slow the pace considerably now, doing the next few exercises in half-time so that you really get the most out of them. If you find the movement awkward or uncomfortable, or have problems with your lower back or knees, place your hands on your thighs for support, or

continue without the use of the bench. Wide, smooth squats are an excellent way to tone up the thighs and buttocks anyway, but still make sure you follow the guidelines below when it comes to foot position and posture. And if you are going to execute them using your bench, it should not be any higher than eight inches so that you don't twist your back.

Stand facing your platform with your feet about twice hip width apart, feet pointing slightly outward for balance and knees soft. Your spine and neck should be lengthened and as always, your stomach and buttocks tucked in with your pelvis tilted forward. Keep your hands on your hips for now — we will add something here when you've got the movement right.

Slowly squat up and down in a smooth

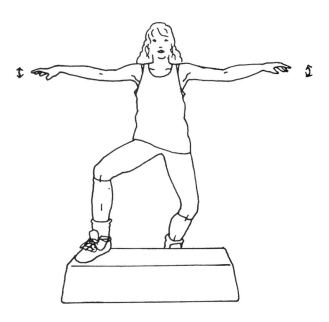

The slow half-step squat — with the straight-arm pulse

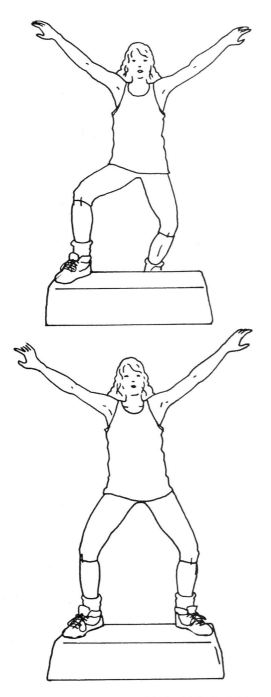

motion which takes two counts to go down and two to rise again, squeezing up through your buttocks to push yourself upward and making sure that you never bend your knees lower than 90 degrees or lock them out on the way up. As always, your knees should be travelling over your feet – try and keep your weight centred.

On the count of four, step up with your right foot as if going into the V-step, but instead of actually stepping up on to the board, hold it in the halfway position – with your right foot at the far right-hand end of the bench and your left still on the floor – and gently squat up and down there four times, once more taking two beats to lower yourself and two beats to come up again. Make sure that you don't arch your back and that your knees are still directly over your feet. Your weight should still be centred – so don't lean away from your leading leg – and, as for all squatting movements, make sure you keep your chest well lifted and press down through your heels so that there is no pressure on your lower back and knees.

Bring your right foot down again, squat gently on the floor four times, and then, maintaining the same slow beat, repeat the whole thing on the other side.

The Slow Full-Step Squat

Begin the slow squat again, but this time complete the V-step, squatting twice this time with your right foot on the bench, twice actually on top of the bench, twice with your right foot stepping down and twice on the floor again – each squat taking four counts every time. So squeeze those buttocks, suck that stomach in and really feel your thighs work. Tap down with the left and repeat the movement on the other side. Again, place your hands on your thighs for support if necessary, still maintaining a good straight back.

The slow full-step squat – with the high straight-arm back squeeze

Slow Alternating Side-on Squat

This time stand on top of your bench facing sideways with your feet pointing straight in front of you and hands on your hips. To the same slow beat of the previous exercises, step down wide to your right, landing gently with the ball of the foot first, followed by the heel and rolling down through into the knee in an easy squat. As with the slow half-step squat, squeeze down and up to four slow beats, but this time with a full body lean from the hips so that you feel as if you are going to sit down over your heels. Keep those stomach muscles well pulled in and your back in a good strong line, and as always, make sure that your knees are travelling over your feet.

Repeat the movement four times and bring your right foot back to the centre briefly so that

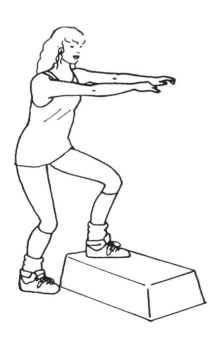

The slow alternating side-on squat — with arms extended

you can step down wide to your left and repeat the exercise on the other side.

For this exercise, simply raise both arms out in front of you at shoulder height to help keep you balanced, with your neck and spine long and straight.

Upper-body Work

This set of arm movements is surprisingly demanding; it is best to make the footwork as simple as possible so that you can concentrate on them fully. They work the shoulders, back, chest and the triceps — basically giving the whole of your upper body a thorough work-over for shape, tone and strength. All should be executed in a slow, controlled manner, resisting the movements all the way but trying to keep the neck and shoulders relaxed.

Start traversing over and back across your bench, tapping down each side and pumping your arms to the music.

Straight-arm Pulse

Now stretch out your arms to the sides at shoulder height, with your palms facing the floor, elbows slightly bent, and shoulders and neck relaxed but with your shoulder blades pressed together as much as possible. Do not arch your back when you do this, though, and think about squeezing the muscles under your arms and across your upper back tight as you pulse your arms slowly and deliberately up and down a couple of inches at your sides, really pushing down against yourself as you lower them and fighting the upward movement as they return to shoulder height.

This movement is small but effective, and

is good to do in combination with the slow squats as your arms pulse twice at every stage of the movement, so helping you to keep your footwork at the right pace.

However, from this basic arm position there are several other variations which you can try:

- **push forward — rotate the palms to face the front and fight against the action all the way**
- **arm circles — think of a piece of string being attached to the fingertips of each hand and stretching out your chest; keep your arms out to your sides.**
- **arm twists — think through your fingertips once more, but this time twisting your wrists forward and back so that your whole arm rotates**

The High Straight-arm Back Squeeze

This next movement squeezes the upper back with your arms raised up above shoulder height.

Raise both arms up to the sides at just above shoulder level so that they are in a wide V-shape. Lift yourself up through your chest, twist your palms so that they face the back of the room, bend your elbows slightly, and, to the same lilting beat that you did your straight-arm pulses, press your arms backward and forward a couple of inches so that you feel your shoulder blades come together and your chest open out. It is a small movement once more, but one that you will notice fairly quickly if you are not used to working these muscles. Again, take care not to arch the back — keep your pelvis well tucked forward and stomach pulled in — and despite working your upper body, try to keep your shoulders as relaxed as possible, with your neck and spine in line.

The Marionette

This arm exercise is tough — but gets excellent results all around the shoulder and neck area.

Draw your arms out to shoulder height at each side as for the straight-arm pulses above, but this time with your palms facing the wall behind you. Now, keeping your elbows high, drop your hands so that they hang loosely as if you were a puppet. Lift and lower through your elbows very slightly. Don't let those elbows drop and concentrate on the action all the time, pulsing gently up and down as you traverse the bench.

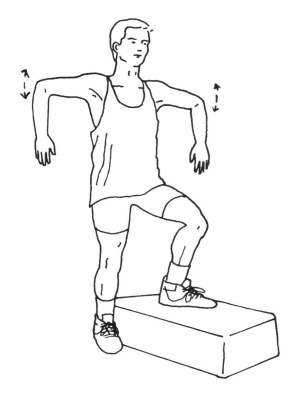

The marionette

The Marionette Back Squeeze

Keeping your elbows at shoulder height, start squeezing your shoulder blades together and apart very slightly so that you really work your upper back. Again, this is a small but challenging movement, so keep those upper arms lifted and pulse your way to a tighter upper body.

The Bent-arm Back Squeeze

To stretch out the chest even more whilst continuing to work the upper back, bring your arms behind you as if you were holding a beach ball against the small of your back. Then, keeping your elbows bent, gently squeeze them together and back so that you really feel the muscles work.

If you have any difficulty with this exercise, lower your hands so that the backs of them rest loosely on your buttocks and try to make a criss-cross movement with them gently behind you, keeping your elbows soft throughout.

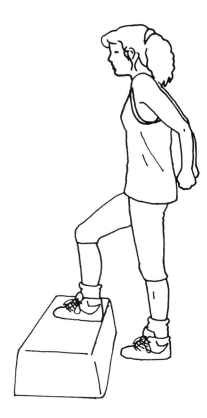

The bent-arm back squeeze

Criss-cross

Now raise both arms out to just below shoulder height in front of you and start to cross them backward and forward in a small controlled motion. Try to squeeze the chest and sides of your body as you do this rather than using your arms, and as always, keep your neck long and shoulders relaxed.

After a while, raise both arms up above your head and continue the movement, resisting the action all the way and isolating the muscles in question.

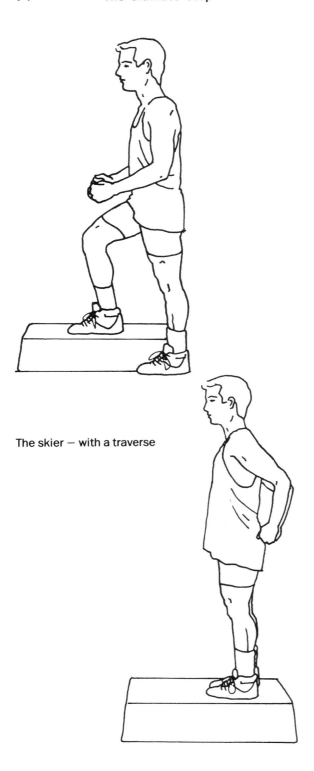

The skier — with a traverse

The Skier

One of my favourites, this really does work and tone up your upper arms and back. So tuck your elbows into your sides with your forearms out to the front as if you are holding on to a pair of ski sticks. From there, squeeze both elbows back until your fists are at your waist and resist the movement as they return to their starting position — simple but effective for toning up your upper arms. Get used to the movement.

The Chest Squeeze

And finally, an exercise which gets me every time. It's a development of the pec deck — and what a development!

Raise your arms into the closed position of the pec deck, with your elbows squeezed together as much as you can at shoulder height and this time with your palms turned so that they are pressed flat against each other. If it helps you maintain this position, lock your fingers together. Then, slowly but surely, press your forearms up and down a couple of inches, squeezing your pecs for all they're worth and really working those upper arms. It won't take long for this to become tiring — believe me!

The Crunching Routine

There's no time like the present to keep those muscles simmering with this final ten-minute routine. Squeeze every fibre, work every movement — and don't be lulled into complacency by their apparent simplicity. Remember — if you don't tone up that body, nobody else will!

Make sure that you are fully warmed up before you start, and lower your bench if you are going to do the squatting movements. Have a sip of water to top up your system — and take a deep breath.

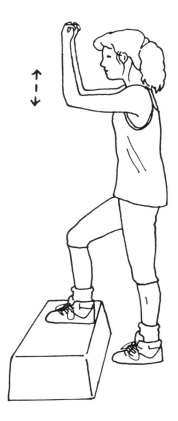

The chest squeeze

1. Start stepping normally, leading with your right leg and pumping your arms vigorously. Tap down and repeat on the other side.

   Repeat 8 times on each side

2. Move into four alternate knee lifts to the front before swinging them gradually to each side, travelling from one end of your bench to the other.

   Continue this throughout the next two arm movements, with four travelling knee lifts for each one.

3. Add the bent-arm back squeeze, pulsing the movement four times with every travelling knee lift.

   Change the arms to the skier.

   And alternate between four travelling knee

lifts with the bent-arm back squeeze and four with the skier four times more.

4. Turn to the centre again and continue with the alternate tap ups. Bring in the marionette back push for four, then the straight marionette for four, and then alternate between each set four more times as above.

5. Continue tapping up and shake your arms out to release any build-up of tension in the shoulders and neck.

   Tap up 8 times

6. Now repeat the pattern, working the pec deck for four steps, the chest squeeze for four, and then alternate between the two sets four times more again.

7. And again, continue this same pattern with the straight-arm pulse and forward push, keeping those arms at shoulder height throughout.

8. Step off your bench this time, shake your arms out again and start squatting gently up and down with your feet about twice hip width apart.

9. On the count of four, work those thighs and buttocks with the slow half-step squat, taking two counts to lower, two counts to raise each time and working alternate sides with four squats to the right, four in the centre and four to the left and so on.

   When you've found your rhythm, introduce the straight-arm back pulse, lifting well out of your chest, flexing the elbows slightly and using your arms to help keep your body-weight centred.

   Repeat each set of four squats
   4 times on each side

10. Develop this into the slow full-step squat, this time doing the high straight-arm back squeeze — and again, sucking in those abdominals tightly to keep your posture upright. Tap down to change the leading leg.
Repeat 4 times on each side

11. March this out into the alternate V-step, pumping those arms.
Repeat 8 times

12. Bring your feet together and start the tap up-tap down leading with the right, pumping your arms vigorously and really working that right thigh. Change the leading leg.
Repeat 8 times on each side

13. Change the leading leg again and add the knee lift every time you step up, introducing the lunge back when you've got into the swing of it. Keep pumping your arms vigorously and change legs.
Repeat 8 times on each side

14. Change the leading leg and step up and down normally with your right as you shuffle to the right-hand end of your bench.

    Tap down to change the leading leg and, on the count of four, begin the crusher — the tap up-tap down step that you practised using the small, straight-legged action out to the side and back — leading with your left and working your left thigh and right buttock.

Repeat 8 times, then add the reps of three, repeating this 4 times, building the reps up to 2 sets of five before winding down again with 2 sets of three reps and finally 4 singles

15. Continue with the normal up-up-down-down step leading with the left, and shuffle over to the other side of your bench, tapping down to repeat the whole thing on the other side.

16. Return to normal stepping on each side to finish off the routine, pumping your arms loosely to begin easing them off.
Repeat 16 times on each side

You probably couldn't face it just now, but next time, why not simply traverse through nos. 1–8 while you work your upper body with some different arm movements, and then introduce the slow alternating side-on squat in combination with some simple lunges? Or what about a sequence of side-on tap up-tap downs interspersed with a few straddles. You see, none of these routines should be fixed for evermore, but once you've got the hang of the various movements involved, you should start thinking about all the different ways you can use them so that you can tailor your workouts to whatever you feel your body needs. In the meantime, though, it's about time you started cooling that body down a bit.

chapter nine

The Cool-down

Easing Out of Your Workout

DESPITE THE FACT that the temptation to head straight for the shower is enormous after a vigorous step workout like that, it is the last thing you should do. You'd never change down from fifth gear to first while belting along the motorway in the fast lane, so why stop dead after exercise?

Cooling down is an essential part of any type of fitness programme and should be taken as seriously as warming up. The dizzy, faint feeling you may experience if you stop too abruptly is simply the result of your blood not having a chance to circulate back from the working muscles to your heart and then brain. But more than that, you are also endangering your heart since it will still be working within your training zone – at as much as 85 per cent of its maximum rate – but with your blood pooling in your legs and unable to return to it since the movement of your muscles is no longer forcing it back. And if nothing else, you'll certainly feel far more sore and uncomfortable over the

next few days than you would if you do cool down and stretch out properly, since your body won't have had a chance to remove the lactic acid which builds up in the working muscles during exercise. In other words, you want to wind your body down, shortening the time it takes to recover from this workout as much as possible and giving yourself a chance to make your next warm-up as comfortable and productive as possible.

So look on your cool-down as a gradual undoing of all that has gone before, building out of the workout just as you built your body into it. It should last at least five minutes, but as long as you don't skimp on the stretches and the process is gradual, there are no hard and fast rules for how you go about it. Just make sure your heart rate has returned to a more normal level before you start stretching, and reread the principles on pp 21–2 to make your movements as safe and effective as possible.

If you are going on to the strengthening exercises in Chapter Ten, lower your heart rate and bring your breathing back to a more normal level following nos. 1–9 below. Then go on to your weight-training work and return to no. 14 below to finish off your whole workout. As before, do the stretches in isolation if it feels more comfortable.

Winding Down

1. Whatever your last step pattern, and whatever your level of intensity, return to the alternate tap up, pumping your arms loosely at your sides.

   Repeat at least 16 times

2. Now add a small kick to the front instead of the tap up, shaking out the arms as well to begin releasing any tension in your upper body.

   Repeat at least 16 times

3. Start leading with your right leg, shrugging your right shoulder forward as you step up, followed by your left, and shrugging them back again in sequence as you step down again. Tap down.

   Repeat at least 8 times on each side

4. Now begin tapping down, rolling both shoulders forward very gently and then backward, keeping your neck relaxed and arms loose.

   Repeat 8 times each way

5. The next time you go to tap down, stay off your bench, marching gently on the spot.

   March for 16 beats

6. Now start tapping the floor gently in front of you, allowing your arms to swing back and forth, following the natural movement of your body.

   Repeat at least 16 times

7. Still tapping out your legs in front of you, take a deep breath and, keeping your lower body moving, draw your arms out to each side in a wide arc, filling your lungs up with air. Hold it there for a few seconds and release it, bringing your arms down again in the process. Now repeat the same action twice more, but this time drawing your arms right up above your head, holding the position for a few seconds before breathing out again and letting your arms come down to your sides once more.

8. Continue tapping your legs out, pumping your arms loosely by your sides.

   Repeat at least 16 times

9. Return to marching on the spot until your heart and lungs are back to normal, although your body is still warm and mobile.

Stretching Out

10. Easing Out the Neck
    Remembering to treat your neck with the utmost care at all times, continue marching on the spot and gently look over towards your right, making sure that your spine is long and that you do not drop your head backward or forward. Hold and return to the centre, carefully looking over towards your left for a few seconds and back to the centre again. Repeat once more on each side.

    Hold for about 10 seconds on each side

11. Stretching Out the Upper Body
    Keeping your lower body moving a little, breathe in deeply as you raise your clasped hands right above your head so that your palms are facing the ceiling, and then breathe out. Hold the position, keeping your shoulders and elbows relaxed and neck

long, again making sure that you don't arch
your back.

Hold for about 10 seconds

12. Stretching Out the Chest

Bring your arms down to your sides once
more and from there, clasp them loosely
behind you. This is the same exercise as
you did in the warm-up, easing your elbows
and shoulder blades together to stretch the
muscles in the chest. As before, don't arch
your back, and keep your elbows soft.

Hold for about 10 seconds and release

13. Stretching Out the Back

Now interlock your fingers in front of you
and raise both arms up to shoulder height,
as if you are holding an elongated beach
ball. Tuck your pelvis well in, keep your
knees soft, and gently pull your shoulder
blades apart so that you feel a good stretch
across the top of your back.

Hold for about 10 seconds and release

*The next four exercises involve lying on your bench
lengthways, so you might like to find a towel or
something to place on top of it to make it a bit more
comfortable. If you are using a milk crate or any other
homemade bench which makes this impractical, simply
do the exercises lying on the floor. Don't just slump
yourself down, though. Sit down carefully and take
care not to twist anything. You may like to put on
a T-shirt if the room's cold.*

14. The Pelvic Tilt

Lie on your back, draw up your knees and
place your feet flat, at a comfortable distance from your buttocks. Now suck the
stomach in tight and press that lower back
firmly downward by tilting your pelvis upward slightly. This is the basic position
that you should be working from for all the

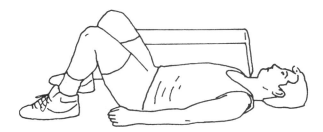
The pelvic tilt

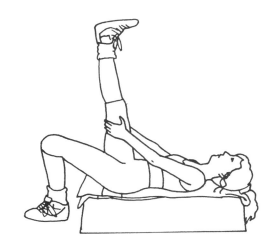
The lying hamstring stretch

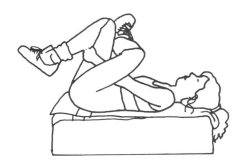
The buttock and hip stretch

following exercises. It is essential that you don't arch your back when you make your moves.

15. **The Lying Hamstring Stretch**

Lie along the top of your bench, with both feet flat on the ground, hip width apart at a comfortable distance from your buttocks. Breathe out deeply so that your whole body is relaxed and make sure that, as with all the abdominal exercises in the following chapter, your pelvis is tilted slightly forward so that your lower back is pressed down flat. Raise your right leg at right angles to your body, supporting it with both hands behind your thigh. And try to straighten the leg as far as is comfortable so that you feel a gentle stretching sensation in the hamstring.

After a few seconds you might like to increase the stretch a fraction by easing your thigh in towards your chest a little more. Keep the leg straight, though, and never force the movement further than is comfortable.

Hold for at least 20 seconds on each side

16. **The Buttock and Hip Stretch**

And now to stretch out those buttocks and hips in a funny-looking position which might take a bit of getting used to.

Start off as for the hamstring stretch above but with both feet flat on the bench about hip width apart. Place your right foot over on to your left thigh, drop your right knee outward and lift your left foot off the bench. Now place your right hand in between your thighs and clasp hold of your left hand underneath your left thigh. Very gently, pull towards your chest until you feel a slight tension around the buttocks. Keep your head and shoulders resting on the bench and your neck relaxed.

Hold for about 10 seconds on each side

17. **Stretching Out the Inner Thighs**

Sit at one end of your bench so that you are facing down it lengthways, with one leg each side.

Sitting well up, with your neck and spine long and straight, extend your legs to each side as wide as is comfortable — you may well feel a slight stretching sensation fairly quickly — so that your feet are flexed and toes pointing up to the ceiling. Support yourself by placing your hands just in front of you — and double-check your position. If you round your back or let your toes point forward, you will not be able to stretch yourself properly.

Now if you want to increase the stretch a little, walk your hands forward a few inches and, keeping your back straight and feet flexed and upright, lean forward from the hips to increase the strength in your inner thighs.

Hold for at least 20 seconds on each side

18. **The Shoulder Stretch — while Releasing Tension in the Calves**

Draw both legs round to the front of your bench, place your feet flat on the floor and, supporting your body weight with both hands

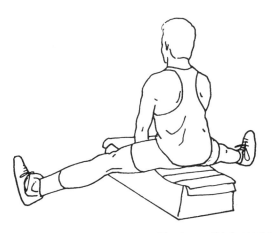

The inner-thigh stretch

on your thighs, stand up, curling up vertebra by vertebra.

Now step up on to your bench once more and stand with your right foot slightly in front of your left. Shift your weight forward on to the right leg, bending it a little and drawing your left foot back so that the heel hangs off the edge of the bench. Don't lean forward from the waist at an exaggerated angle — keep your neck and spine long and chest lifted — and gently push downward on to the left heel until you feel a slight stretch in the calf, keeping the left knee slightly bent. Don't bounce. Keep the pressure even and balanced. And don't overstretch.

When you have got the position, bring the opposite arm — your left — across your body at chest height. Very gently, ease it inward towards your body with your right arm until you feel a gentle stretch in the left shoulder.

Hold for about 10 seconds
then repeat both stretches
on the other side

19. The Triceps Stretch — while Releasing Tension in the Calves

Swap legs again so that you are back easing out the left calf once more, but this time stretch out the right triceps as you do so.

As in the warm-up, raise your right arm and then drop your hand behind your head, keeping your elbow pointing towards the ceiling. Then use your left hand to ease it gently over towards the left until you feel a slight stretching sensation along the underside of your arm.

Hold for about 10 seconds
then repeat both stretches
on the other side

20. The Quadriceps Stretch

Now stand on the floor, centre your weight

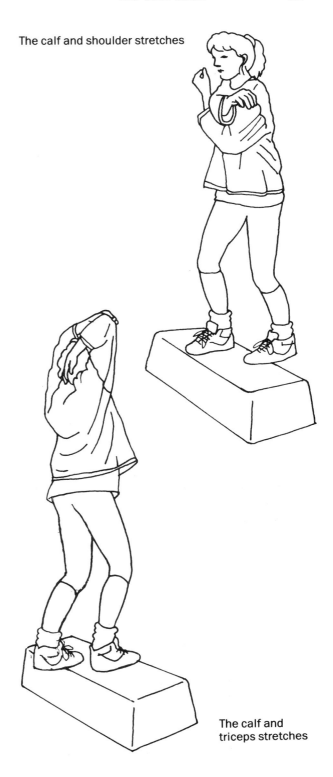

The calf and shoulder stretches

The calf and
triceps stretches

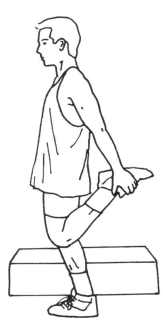

The quadriceps stretch

on your right leg and bring your left foot up towards your buttocks. Keep your knees close together and tilt your pelvis forward so that you feel a slight stretch down the front of your left thigh and hip. Don't lock out your supporting leg though.

Hold for about 10 seconds on each side

You should now be feeling tired, but relaxed and full of energy. So clear away your bench carefully, bending your knees as you pick it up and holding it close into your chest as you carry it off. Well done! You've probably just completed the most invigorating workout of your life.

chapter ten

Abdominals and Others

Adding a Bit of Muscle

WEIGHTS FOR BOYS and aerobics for girls. There's always a comforting ring about fallacies. But benchwork has rewritten the rules when it comes to male aerobics, and it's time to think again about strength training.

The more muscle your body has, the more energy your body can burn up on a daily basis. Strength training is not in itself the most effective way of reducing body fat — although sit-ups may *feel* extremely demanding, the actual energy required for the movement is far less than, say, a quick walk round the block, since you are taking your entire body weight for a stroll with you rather than simply lifting and lowering your top half a few inches off the floor. But strength training can change your body shape, proportion and composition, leaving you far better toned. Also, the stronger you are, the less easily you'll tire, not only in step but in other everyday activities — everything from carrying the shopping home to a good night's sex — because you will be able

to process and store energy that much more efficiently. On top of that, the more muscle you have, the less likely you are to sustain stress-related injuries since your skeletal frame will be better supported, your internal organs better protected and your posture better, full stop. Moreover, cross training which incorporates benchwork into an interval-training programme where, for example, you step for three minutes, strength train for three etc., reduces the risk of so-called 'overuse syndrome', where injuries develop as a result of working your muscles and joints in one particular way too often. Then think about the longer-term view for a moment — weight-bearing exercise has been shown to play a part in delaying and reducing the chances of osteoporosis (brittle bone disease) — and I think you'll agree that the arguments for continuing to work through this chapter are mounting up rapidly. And if you've just invested in a bench of your own, it's also nice to know all the different ways you can make use of it — if fluorescent moulded plastic coffee tables aren't your idea of chic interior design, maybe.

Remember, it takes a lot more than a few triceps dips to make a Mr Universe, and muscle does not turn into instant blubber the moment you stop your exercises. So look on the positive side to weight-training and enjoy your new-found strength.

Jargon of the Gym

A few principles to think about when strength training.

- **Resistance — it takes effort to get results. Whether working against your own resistance or increasing the demand by adding extra weight, your body responds because you are putting your muscles under stress. Reps without effort get you nowhere.**
- **Overload — pushing yourself slightly beyond your normal work capacity so that your body is forced to adapt by using more muscle fibres with every rep, so making them thicker and stronger. This can be adapted by either training for endurance (with a relatively low amount of weight and a lot of reps) or for strength (with a lot of weight and only a few reps). It is the latter which produces the classic bodybuilding dimensions.**
- **Technique — a word you're probably sick of by now, but one which applies equally to strength-training exercises as to benchwork. As in Chapter Eight, control is the key, working the given muscle or muscles in a smooth, slow action. Momentum is out.**

Adding Some Weight

As we have seen, this is the part of your step training programme which allows you to

incorporate handweights into some of the exercises safely. Although small 1.5 lb weights may well be sufficient for now — or, indeed, a small plastic bottle filled with water or a tin of food, maybe — you can increase these to 2 lb, 3 lb and so on as your capacity improves. Still:

1. **Never warm up or cool down using weights.**

2. **If they are the hand-held variety rather than wrist bands, avoid squeezing them too tightly or you could make your blood pressure rise. Also make sure that your wrist and forearm remain in line. Don't allow your hand to flex either upward or downward.**

3. **Always make sure you are familiar with the given movements before you start adding to the resistance.**

4. **Make doubly sure that momentum doesn't swing your arms about, as you could easily pull a muscle or joint too far.**

5. **As always, never lock your joints out — in this case your knees and elbows.**

6. **Stop if you feel any real discomfort.**

7. **And an obvious point to conclude with, but if you are at all unsure about your suitability to use handweights in this way — if, say, you are pregnant, have high blood pressure or maybe have problems with your joints — take medical advice.**

Of course, you can always increase the workload of the first two groups of exercises — the hip and thigh trio, and the all-fours — by looping one of those long elastic training bands around your ankles. A word of caution, though. If you wish to walk away from them with all your skin still intact, make sure that band and flesh do not meet. Wedge the elastic into a fold in your socks. And try out the exercises before rushing off to the shops. They are quite intense enough without the extra resistance – believe me.

And So to Work

Unlike the other exercises in this book, this last batch should all be treated independently and are not linked together in any kind of routine.

> 'Make the muscles do the work in a steady up-down rhythm. [They] should be raised and lowered at the same speed. Your reps should almost be done in slow motion, *finding* the fibres along the way. Think of pouring molasses from a jar on a winter's day . . .'
>
> Bob Paris, *Beyond Built*

Try and repeat each exercise:

- **three times with one slow beat to lift, one slow beat to lower – two counts in all**
- **three times taking three slow beats to lift and three to lower – six counts in all**
- **and three times to the two-beat count again.**

Don't worry if you can't manage this straightaway. And don't be smug if this is far too easy for you. Adapt the number accordingly, with a maximum of about a minute spent on each one.

I like to do a few of these exercises – especially the abdominal work – at the end of my benchwork routine, once my pulse has returned to a more normal level but before I've cooled down too much. However, there's nothing to stop you doing them independently of your workouts. Always make sure that you are fully warmed up before you start, though, and ease out your neck, back and chest with the three stretches below before finishing off with the remaining stretches on pp 79–82. As before, do the exercises and stretches on your bench or on the floor, depending on which is more comfortable. Use a towel or mat for additional cushioning if you wish.

The Hip and Thigh Trio

Sit down carefully on the end of your bench with your knees loosely together, place both hands behind you holding on to each side of your bench with your elbows soft, and lean back a little so that your body weight is supported.

Sitting Leg Raise

Extend your right leg in front of you so that the heel is resting lightly on the floor. Gently lift it up until it is parallel to the ground and lower it again slowly so that the heel is just above the floor – not touching it. You'll feel the muscles in your right thigh almost immediately – so repeat the movement and really concentrate on strengthening those thighs.

Repeat following the 2-6-2 count

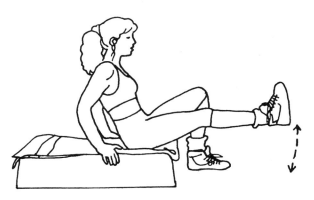

The sitting leg raise

If you do have any back problems, sit right back on your bench so that both legs are supported fully, arms behind you as before and lift and lower your legs a couple of inches and no more.

Then draw your right knee in towards your chest and maintain this position for the sitting thigh push and raise.

Sitting Thigh Push and Raise

Flex your foot and slowly push it out in front of you until the knee is almost locked out before drawing it back in again, still resisting the movement at every stage. Repeat, and then hold that position with your knee drawn into your chest, carefully dropping your right knee out to the side. It's time to focus on that inner thigh, so this time lift and lower your flexed right foot slightly across your body so that you can really feel the inside of your thigh work.

Repeat following the 2-6-2 count
and change sides

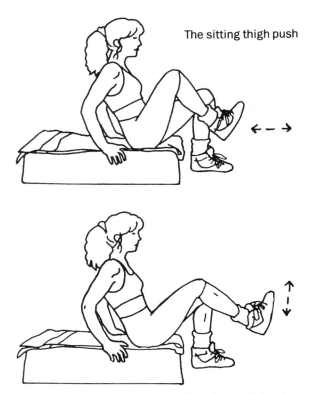

The sitting thigh push

←–→

The sitting thigh raise

Remember – all these can be intensified by looping one of those long, workout rubber bands around both ankles, increasing the resistance considerably.

All Fours

Now kneel down on top of your bench or all fours, or, if you find it more comfortable resting on your elbows. It's time to concentrate on the backs of the thighs and buttocks a bit more, balancing out the thigh trio above and improving the power of your bench-stepping.

All Fours Buttocks and Hamstring Squeeze

Keeping your stomach well pulled in and neck and spine in line, extend your right leg so that it is parallel to the floor, making quite sure that you don't arch your back. Very slowly, lift your leg a couple of inches, feeling the contraction in your right buttock and hamstring, and lower it again gently.

Repeat, following the 2-6-
and hold that positio

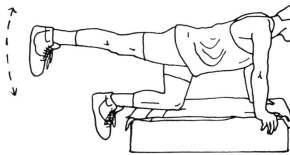

The all-fours buttocks and hamstring squeeze

All Fours Leg Curl and Buttock Crusher

From there, curl your heel slowly up toward your buttocks, squeezing the back of your thigh as you practised in the standing position and

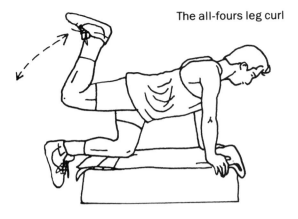

The all-fours leg curl

times, and don't allow your thigh to drop down too far towards the bench.

Repeat following the 2-6-2 count and change sides

Again, looping a long workout band round both ankles when you do these exercises will increase the demand made on your muscles considerably. Personally, I'd practise a while first!

The Back

Having a little lie-down after the last movements, stretch out on your stomach. It's time to work your back — an easy part to forget since most people are only concerned with the areas that they can see when standing in front of a full-length mirror. However, because many people experience back trouble, you should be sensible about approaching this exercise, and stop at the slightest warning twinge.

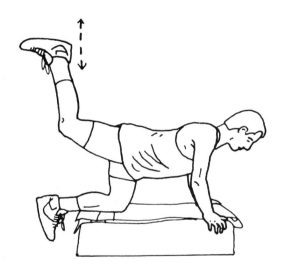

The all-fours buttock crusher

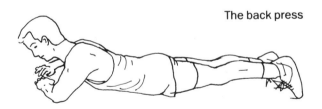

The back press

keeping that stomach well pulled in so that you don't strain your lower back. Uncurl it again, making sure that your thigh is still parallel to the floor and repeat so that you finish with your heel curled inward. Hold it there again . . . and to complete this gruesome trio, with the sole of your right foot pointing directly up to the ceiling, squeeze the right buttock so that you lift and lower your thigh a couple of inches each way. Your back should be kept flat at all

Back Press

Rest your chin on your hands in front of you with your elbows pointing out to the sides. Suck your stomach in and, tilting your pelvis forward to avoid overstressing your back, push gently upward from your forearms until your chin is a couple of inches off the ground. Keep your neck and spine in line by watching the floor all the time, and slowly lower again.

Lying flyes

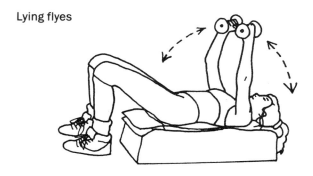

Never push yourself right up on to your hand — a couple of inches is all it needs.

Repeat following the 2-6-2 count

Pectoral Power

Now for a couple of exercises which will strengthen and define your chest and shoulders enormously – as well as help women redress the effects of gravity in this area. So practise each exercise to perfect your technique, and then introduce a bit of weight.

Lying Flyes

You should be familiar with the flye movement by now and know what muscular sensation you are looking for in your pectorals.

Raise your arms up at chest height in front of you, palms facing each other and about shoulder width apart. The elbows should never be locked out but kept slightly flexed. Now slowly draw your arms out and down to either side of your body in a wide semicircle until you feel a gentle stretch across your chest. Your palms should still be facing each other and your elbows slightly bent to protect them when you add handweights. Squeeze the pectorals and slowly return your hands to the starting position through the same wide controlled arc – squeezing them a fraction more in the middle just for good measure – and always making sure that the small of your back remains flat against the bench.

Repeat following the 2-6-2 count

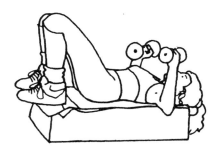

Lying Chest Press

Now draw both hands in towards your chest so that they are a comfortable distance apart, knuckles pointing straight up to the ceiling. Exhale and push your hands upward at right

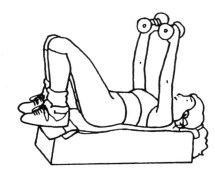

The lying chest press

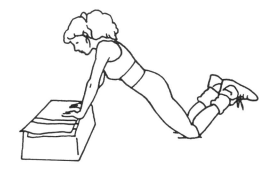

angles to your body so that your elbows are almost locked out but not quite. Inhale and bring them in once more and repeat, as always making sure that your pelvis is tipped slightly upward so that your lower back stays firmly planted on your bench. Concentrate on squeezing those shoulders and working that chest.

Repeat following the 2-6-2 count

Push-ups

And so to my *bête noire*, push-ups — killing for arms, shoulders, back . . . in fact, excellent for the whole of the upper body! Kneel down in front of your bench and reach forward to hold on to it with your arms about shoulder width apart. Gradually support yourself on your arms, never fully extending your elbows. Cross your feet if it feels more comfortable, keep your buttocks sticking out a bit and suck the stomach in to protect your lower back, pulling upward from your pelvis in a strong line which keeps your spine and neck long. Then gently lower yourself towards the bench as far as you can. That's the easy bit. Now squeeze those shoulders, arms and chest, exhale and push yourself gradually upward to your starting position, making sure that you don't arch your back or lock your elbows out.

Repeat following the 2-6-2 count as capable!

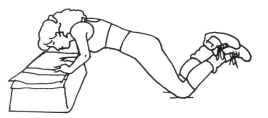

The push-up

Now, keeping your hands on top of the bench still, lower your feet to the floor and gently shift your body weight backward over them — never pulling back too far but just giving yourself enough space to stretch out your upper body. You should be looking straight down to the floor with your neck and spine in line. Hold this relaxed position for a few seconds.

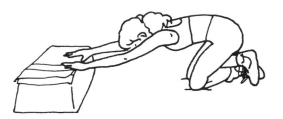

The push-up back stretch

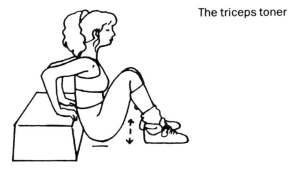

The triceps toner

The Arms

It's time to continue working those arms a bit more now, concentrating on the two major muscle groups — the biceps and the triceps. You may well find that the 2-6-2 repetition is too low for you here, so increase accordingly.

Triceps Toner

This is one of my favourite exercises because, unlike push-ups, I can do it relatively easily. So sit on the side of your bench with your hands holding on to the edge and both your fingers and your feet pointing straight ahead, feet flat on the floor about hip width apart. Shift your weight forward so that you are supporting yourself on your arms — keeping your elbows soft, of course — and slowly lower your buttocks towards the floor. Try not to collapse and sit right down. Stay a couple of inches above the ground and then raise yourself upward again, without locking your elbows out at the top. Keep your buttocks close to the bench, your spine and neck straight and keep looking forward.

It may take some time to build up the strength in your triceps, but when you can comfortably do about a dozen of these, increase the intensity by drawing your feet out further from the bench in front of you.

Repeat following the 2-6-2 count

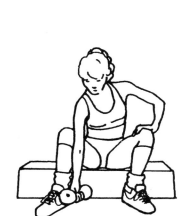

Sitting Bicep Curl

And to balance this, sit on your bench with your legs apart, feet flat on the floor in a comfortable position. As always, your upper body should be relaxed but strong. Rest your right elbow just inside your right knee to keep your upper arm still, and drop your forearm towards the floor. Squeeze your biceps a fraction to find that contraction and then slowly curl your fore-

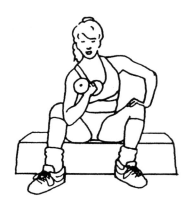

The sitting bicep curl

arm upward towards your shoulder, exhaling as you do so until your hand is at shoulder height facing you. Lower it again under control, swapping arms after the desired number of reps.

Repeat following the 2-6-2 count

The Abdominals

And so to the area which seems to draw the gaze like a magnet the moment you see a full-length mirror. The stomach, the guts, the belly, midriff: call it what you like, most people would do almost anything to get it into shape.

And most people know at least a couple of exercises to tone it all up — indeed, there sometimes seems to be an endless supply of different movements on offer. The ones below are among the easiest to master, though, providing a couple of variations on two basic themes — the curl and the crunch. Don't attempt to do all of them in one go, but pick out one or two each time — a straight up-and-down movement and a twisting movement maybe, so that you work both the front of the stomach and the waist a bit too — and gradually develop the strength and tone of this whole area. If nothing else, the added strength here will help your posture enormously while you step — and so help avoid injury.

It is essential to squeeze your abdominal muscles as hard as you can during every exercise, though. Nobody else is going to do this for you, and it's not good enough simply to wrench your head and shoulders forward in a wild exaggerated momentum-driven movement. So contract those abdominals to make your shoulders lift, and control the movement on the way down too.

Repeat each exercise at least ten times — including some slow movements which take three counts to rise

and three to fall as you have done for all the preceding exercises.

Abdominal Warm-up

From your pelvic tilt position (see p 79), place your hands lightly behind the nape of your neck with your elbows pointing upward. Suck your stomach in, and curl your shoulders forward a couple of inches while at the same time drawing your right knee up towards your chest. Squeeze the abdominals in the middle and slowly release, controlling your descent all the way before repeating the movement with your left leg. Continue with this action a few times before beginning the abdominal work in earnest. It is a gentle way of preparing your stomach for the work ahead.

Repeat about 10 times

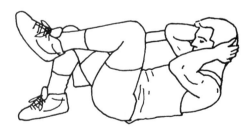

The abdominal warm-up

Curl-ups — Arms Extended

Using your arms for nothing more than balance, place them lightly on your thighs about half-way up. Keep your chin lifted and suck your abdominals in tightly, using them alone — and not your shoulders — to curl slowly up from the top of your spine, raising your shoulder blades no more than a couple of inches so that your hands lightly touch your knees. Remember — this is a

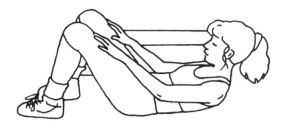

The curl-up — with arms extended

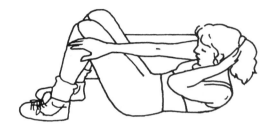

The curl-up — with alternate arms

small movement. It is not the distance you travel that matters, but the amount you squeeze.

Although the natural reaction is to breathe in sharply when you do this, try to breathe out every time your head rises as it will help your abdominals to contract.

Repeat about 10 times, or more if you can

Curl-ups — Alternate Arms

From there, place your right hand behind your head and slide your left hand across to the outside of your right knee, to work the side of your stomach a bit more. This time, though, take one count to lift, one to squeeze your arm over, one to come back to the centre and one to lower again.

Repeat about 10 times to each side

Curl-ups — Hands Behind Head

Now place both hands lightly behind your head with your elbows pointing out and chin lifted, and continue with your curl-ups as before.

Repeat about 10 times,
more if you can

Pulses

This time, *pulse* the movement so that the action takes half the time — just one beat to lift and lower. Your body position will be slightly modified as you begin with your shoulders curled up off the bench and push forward and back from there, never allowing your muscles to relax. You will therefore probably start feeling it fairly quickly — especially if you really are squeezing your stomach hard throughout — so don't overdo it!

Repeat about 10 times

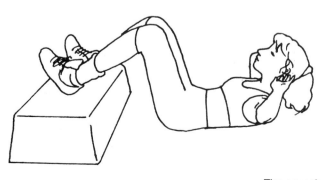

The crunch

The Crunch

With your heels resting gently on top of your bench and a good clean right-angle bend at the knees, place both hands behind your head with your elbows pointing out to the side. Once more curl up and down, really feeling the 'crunch' as the muscles contract – don't just go through the motions.

Repeat about 10 times,
more if you can

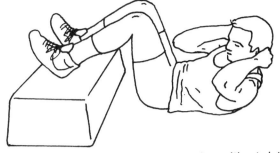

The crunch – with a twist

The Crunch – with a Twist

Add a twist this time as you raise your shoulders, so that your right elbow meets your left knee, your left elbow meets your right knee. Again, work from the 'pulse' position, with your shoulders lifted off the floor, twisting in a smooth and continuous movement which keeps the muscles working.

Repeat about 10 times,
more if you can

The Raised Leg Crunch

For a more demanding exercise which might take a little practice, raise your legs slightly with your feet together. Bring your right hand from behind your head and reach upward towards your feet and then lower it again, squeezing at the point of greatest contraction.

Now reach across your body to the outside of your left leg and, shoulders lifted once again, repeat the movement. Swap hands and practise these movements on the other side too.

Repeat about 10 times,
more if you can

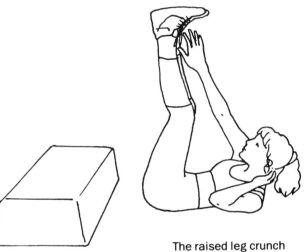

The raised leg crunch

The Crunch – with a Pelvic Lift

As you can probably feel, the first batch of exercises focused mainly on the upper abdominal

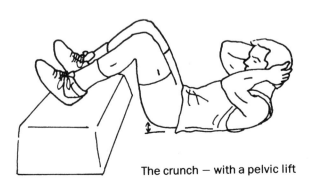

The crunch – with a pelvic lift

The reverse curl

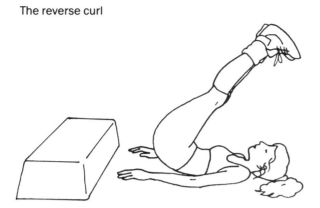

The lower-back stretch

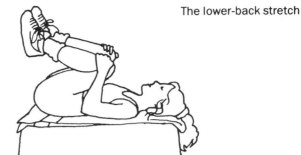

muscles and those down the sides. The lower abs are a different matter – and quite a difficult one too. So go back to the crunch position (p 79), except this time, try and squeeze your lower abdominal muscles as well so that you not only raise your shoulders a couple of inches off the ground but your buttocks too.

Repeat about 10 times,
more if you can

Reverse Curl

Finally, with your feet raised once more as for the raised leg crunch and with your hands supporting your neck or by your sides for balance, slowly and carefully curl your hips a few inches off the floor by contracting your lower abdominals again. Release them and repeat, resisting the temptation to push yourself up with your arms.

Repeat about 10 times,
more if you can

Lower Back Stretch

Now draw both knees carefully into your chest, hugging them tight to release any build-up of tension in the back.

Winding Down

And so to a few stretches which will gradually ease your upper body out after all the abdominal and strengthening work. Reread the dos and don'ts of stretching in Chapter Five (pp 21–2) if necessary, and use these last moments to wind down before going back to p 80 for the hamstring, hip, inner thigh and calf stretches at the very end of your cool-down.

Easing Out the Neck

It is very easy for tension to build up in the neck area during this type of work, so stretch it out gently with this simple exercise.

Lie on the bench or floor with your knees bent, feet placed flat and about hip width apart, with the small of your back pushed well down and your pelvis tilted slightly up. Your spine should be lengthened and straight, with a good long neck, and you should let your arms rest loosely by your sides. Breathe in deeply and, as you exhale, look gently over to your right and hold for a few seconds. Breathe in again, returning your head to the centre, and repeat the movement on the other side, never overstraining the neck, but keeping it long and relaxed throughout.

Easing Out the Chest and Upper Body

Still maintaining the same body position, take another deep breath, and draw your hands out to either side in a slow, wide arc until they are just above shoulder height. Keep your palms facing the ceiling and gently ease your arms downward and slightly backward so that you open up your ribcage and feel a stretching sensation right across your chest. Hold for a few seconds and relax, exhaling as you bring your arms back to the starting position.

Inhale deeply once again, this time drawing your arms outward and right up over your head and back a fraction so that you feel your whole spine lengthening slightly, easing away any build-up of tension in your upper body. Hold as before and exhale once more, bringing your hands down to your sides again. Repeat this movement one more time, making sure that the small of your back remains well pressed down on to your bench.

Now return to no. 15 on p 80 to finish off your stretches in the cooling-down section. You are now only minutes away from that steaming hot shower. So hang in there for these last four stretches and try not to head straight for the biscuit tin when you've finished.

chapter eleven

High-energy Eating

Food to Fuel an Active Life

IF THERE'S ONE subject guaranteed to attract attention it's food. From magazines to TV programmes, gourmet cuisine to the weekly shop, this multi-million-pound industry is devoted to the sole cause of eating more, while current ideals in fashion and beauty dictate that we refrain. And where does this leave us? Right in the middle, spending money trying to do both.

So if scales are your anathema and the very mention of the word 'diet' conjures up images of guilt, self-sacrifice and deprivation, read on. This is not a diet chapter but a few words on *eating*. There are plenty of other books providing complicated tables and eating plans for weight loss, if that's what you're really after. All you'll find here is a positive, healthy approach to food which allows you to enjoy the sensation of a well-filled stomach while providing abundant energy to fuel your new, more active lifestyle.

Back to Basics

The good news is that the basis of a normal healthy diet is very similar to one designed to support an energetic lifestyle. Both involve moderation, variety and wholesomeness:

- **moderation — to make sure that you don't eat more than your body needs, since an excess of anything will be turned straight into body fat**
- **variety — to ensure you receive a good balanced diet with appropriate quantities of the big three — protein, fat and carbohydrate — not to mention vitamins, minerals and water**
- **wholesomeness — as a rule of thumb, the more a given food is processed, the less nutritional value it has. Therefore you should aim at, say, wholemeal bread rather than white, fresh orange juice rather than carbonated cans and so on.**

If all you do is bear those points in mind when you choose your foods, you're already well on the way to healthier eating. But what exactly does this mean in terms of eating for energy?

Fuels for Exercise

The way energy is stored and used in your body represents the stepping stone between what you eat and how well you perform. It is provided through your food in three main ways, protein, fat and carbohydrate – although a fourth, more entertaining form, alcohol, should perhaps be mentioned, since fitness and a good night out on the town are not mutually exclusive. However, while alcohol may contribute massively to your overall calorie intake, it cannot be used as a direct source of energy by your exercising muscles since its breakdown is only carried out in your liver. And just for reference, a good Saturday morning step workout is very definitely *not* the ultimate hangover cure. The diuretic effect of alcohol can play havoc with any attempts you make to keep your fluid levels up, while the rhythmic marching up and down can leave your head thumping.

Of the more stable three, though, fat and carbohydrate are the front runners when it comes to exercise, and exactly how much energy is derived from each depends on the nature of your activity. Carbohydrates are your primary source, being converted into glucose – blood sugar – when eaten and either used up immediately by the brain and muscles, or stored in limited amounts as glycogen in the muscles and liver as a readily available supply of energy during physical exertion. Roughly speaking, carbohydrates are responsible for the first 5–15 minutes of aerobic exertion, after which point the body starts using its carbohydrate stores in conjunction with body fat – a far greater potential source of energy – irritatingly great for a lot of people.

The building blocks of fat, the fatty acids, are released from the stores beneath the skin, and the muscles start burning up a mixture of the two, eking out the limited glycogen reserves to make them last longer. While the use of glycogen is largely specific to the muscles being worked, free fatty acids can be derived from anywhere in the body. This is the reason you can't 'spot reduce' fat – that is, burn it away specifically around, say, your stomach.

So why doesn't the body utilize its fat stores as the major source of energy right from the start? For the simple reason that you can't burn fat fast enough to supply the necessary amount. Run out of glycogen and you literally run out of energy. Hence the experience of 'hitting the wall' towards the end of an endurance race. However, when you train more often and your energy demands are higher, your body adapts. It increases the amount of fat used in the initial stages of your exercise so that your energy levels can be maintained for longer and your fat reserves can be burned up more readily.

And protein? Only when you've been exercising for two or three hours – at the very end of a marathon, for instance – and your carbohydrate stores have been depleted, may protein be called upon for energy. Even then, however, it will only contribute about 10 per cent to the overall energy cost.

Supply and Demand

So whatever the activity, some carbohydrate will be used for energy in the form of glycogen, fat provides a secondary store and protein a last resort. It therefore makes sense that your food should reflect this balance. If you want to delay the point at which fatigue sets in during training, it stands to reason that you should start off with your glycogen stores fully topped up, making carbohydrates your major food source — comprising at least 55–65 per cent of the energy in your diet.

A Complex Question

With about 4 calories per gramme, dietary carbohydrates are made up of various combinations of carbon, hydrogen and oxygen to produce so-called 'simple' and 'complex' carbohydrates. While both have a similar ability to fuel your muscles, the difference in their construction affects the way that their energy is released, not to mention the fact that the sources of each have different abilities to nourish our bodies with vitamins and minerals.

Solid and Sustaining

Complex carbohydrates — 'starchy' fibrous foods like potatoes, pulses, pasta, wholegrain cereals and bread — are made from long chains of sugars all joined together. They're the foods that dieters have traditionally avoided like the plague because they have always been considered 'fattening'. But it's time to give them their due because they're the ideal nourishment for weightwatchers and athletes alike:

- **they aren't high in calories — one large slice of wholemeal bread has only 70-odd calories (whereas the butter on top — ⅓ oz or 10 g — adds as many calories again)**
- **they're low in fat — less than 2 calories come from unsaturated fat in 8 oz (225 g) of potatoes**
- **they're bulky — filling you up quickly, leaving less space for other, more fattening options**
- **they're excellent food for exercise — being absorbed into the bloodstream slowly, stabilizing your blood sugar (blood glucose)**

- **levels over a long period, meaning you have more energy more of the time**
- **they're nutrient dense — rich in a variety of vitamins, minerals and protein**
- **and they're rich in fibre, the plant material which is indigestible by man and which sweeps out waste from the digestive system.**

Looked at like this, it becomes clear that the bad reputation complex carbohydrates have inherited stems not from the foods in themselves, but from the way that they're cooked and served. So resist the sour cream on your baked potato and the slabs of butter and cheese on your bread, go for a tomato-based sauce on your pasta rather than a creamy one, and ditch the mayo — always! It simply doesn't make sense to smother a nutritious salad with fat-filled dressings when there's yoghurt or lemon juice on offer.

Complex carbohydrates are not fattening — they're fuel, the real staff of life.

Simply Sweet

As their name suggests, the simple sugars which form the basis of things like honey and table sugar have a relatively simple construction and are quickly converted into blood glucose by the body. You get an initial surge of energy as your blood sugar levels soar and then, once the insulin in your body has balanced the levels again, you can get that all-too-familiar slump. That's not to say that all sweets and confectionery are out. Far from it. If your energy demands are high and the bulky nature of the complex carbohydrates at the heart of your eating becomes too much, a good old-fashioned bar of chocolate makes an ideal addition to your diet, especially after training — although it should be said that cereal bars and, even better, fresh or dried fruit will give the same results while providing you with additional vitamins, minerals and fibre and little fat. In other words, try and pick the more wholesome snacks if you really need a boost, and keep the 'empty' processed foods as treats.

Fat of the Land

In terms of calories, fats are expensive. Be it animal or vegetable, saturated or unsaturated, a single gramme is loaded with 9 calories of energy, a single teaspoon with about 36 — that is, over twice the amount in carbohydrates. But cutting them out completely is definitely not the answer. Your body needs dietary fats since they provide the fat-soluble vitamins A, D, E and K, while the likes of vegetable oils provide the essential free fatty acids needed for the production of several hormones and maintaining healthy cell membranes. So treat fats with care — about 20–25 per cent of your total energy intake is more than sufficient — and try to watch which fats you eat. An overload of saturated fats — those found in animal products like full-fat milk, cheese and cream, and fatty meat like streaky bacon, mince, sausages, pâté and pork pies — may raise blood cholesterol levels and thus increase the chances of heart disease.

Choose low-fat dairy products such as semi-skimmed milk and cottage cheese, reduced-fat cheddars and Quark; head for the lean cuts of red meat, chicken, fish and pulses, and watch out for the hidden saturated fats in processed cakes, pastry, biscuits, sweets and chocolate. Similarly, a few culinary adjustments might not go amiss. Why deep fry when you can stir fry? Why fry when you can grill? Why not steam your fish next time or bake it in foil in the oven? And how about skinning those chicken legs or scooping the fat off your gravy? Keeping your dietary fat down will not cramp your culinary style, but it will help to enhance your athletic ability — and your health!

Protein and Performance

Protein forms as essential a role in the sports diet as it does in any other. Since it is fundamental for all tissue growth and repair, and there is more of it in the body than any other substance except water, it might, therefore, seem natural to assume that a diet rich in protein offers the perfect recipe for athletic prowess. Thus if you eat more of it, your performance will improve. Or will it?

Go into any sports shop and you will see the vast array of power breakfasts, protein builders, amino acid supplements, branch-chain amino acid compounds and the like, all with the promise of peak performance, all offering a shortcut to achievement. There is one school of thought which rightly points out that the daily recommended allowance of each nutrient in the diet takes no account of the fact that athletes in training make far higher demands of their body and so may need higher quantities of these nutrients. Yet research shows that muscle mass — and hence the body's ability to store and process energy — is only substantially increased by appropriate exercise, and that an increase in muscular activity does not necessarily demand a comparable increase in protein intake. Raw eggs and slabs of red meat are not the muscle behind the weights room after all, and the standard recommended 1.0–1.5 g of protein per kilo of body weight — approximately 15–20 per cent of the energy in your whole diet — will suffice, adequately catered for in a normal well-balanced diet. After all, an excess of protein in the body is treated in exactly the same way as an excess of any other food. It is turned straight into body fat.

Garnish your Meals

Try looking on the protein you eat as a garnish rather than the focus of your meals, and, as with everything else, pay a bit more attention to which sources of protein you choose, since the more conventional high-protein foods are usually high in fats as well.

Take dairy products. Rich in calcium and vitamin B_2, which help to build strong bones (and possibly to prevent osteoporosis), they are an excellent source of protein, especially if, like me, you always seem to be eating on the run. However, as we have already seen, they also provide you with a lot of saturated fat that you could well do without. So again choose low-fat dairy products, go for lean varieties of meat – like chicken or turkey (without the skin) – and don't forget about the abundance of vegetable-based proteins found in pulses like kidney beans, split peas, lentils and soya beans.

It is worth remembering, though, that most animal products are considered 'complete' since they contain a relatively high proportion of the essential amino acids that your body cannot produce for itself, while vegetable sources may well be low in one or more of these essential amino acids and are sometimes referred to as 'incomplete' – only a concern if you go without any animal protein in your daily diet at all. A chunky bean stew with rice provides a good nutrient-dense plateful, though, and most people pad out their nut roasts with breadcrumbs for economic reasons anyway, without even considering the balance of cereals and nuts which this provides. And what else can baked beans sit on than good old toast?

Remember – for a sustaining diet which will keep your fat levels down but your energy levels high, it is the complex carbohydrates which should make up most of your diet, then the fats and then the proteins.

Vitamins and Minerals

Although often thought of as the boosters from the bottles, these dietary essentials can be obtained from a variety of sources – although it should be said that food processing can often destroy them. Minerals, like calcium, iron and sodium, and vitamins all perform their individual tasks in the body's structure and functioning, and there may well be some instances – in childhood, adolescence, pregnancy and old age, for example – when you are advised by your doctor to take vitamin or mineral supplements for medical reasons. But chomping your way indiscriminately through the contents of those small brown bottles in the hope that this will lead to a healthier, more productive life could, in fact, lead to nutritional imbalances in your body. As long as you consume foods from all four main food groups –

grains and cereals
dairy products
fruit and veg – including potatoes
and proteins – animal and vegetable

– supplementation is generally unnecessary. So, for instance, if red meat and offal are inappropriate sources of iron for you, there are always green leafy vegetables like spinach (also full of vitamin C) – not to mention wholegrain cereals and bread, oily fish, pulses and nuts, with a handful of dried fruit such as figs and apricots for a little variety. And for the vegans among you, don't forget the B_{12} fortified soya products, spreads and breakfast cereals to compensate for this one deficiency in your diet.

Fluid

Now for the substance which makes up about 70 per cent of your body – water. You'll only last a couple of days without this simple combination of hydrogen and oxygen whereas you can last a great deal longer without food. When it comes to exercising hard, fluid is of crucial concern because of its role in regulating your body temperature.

Surprisingly, perhaps, only about 20–25 per cent of the energy produced from digesting carbohydrates and fats is actually used to contract your muscles and propel you around. The rest? Lost as heat – and when you exercise, your body produces vast amounts of heat as it burns your energy reserves away. However, to prevent an ever-spiralling body temperature, this heat is dissipated by a process called vasodilation, whereby the flow of blood to the skin is increased so that it travels nearer to the cooling outside air. Hence the rosy glow in your cheeks. Then, if your body still can't take the heat, phase two is introduced – sweat, cooling you down through evaporation and enabling you to perform intense physical exertion for prolonged amounts of time.

As sweat is nothing more than a dilute version of blood, your body will lose not only water but, to a far lesser degree, so-called electrolytes – primarily salt. A small decrease in the latter does not really cause any problems in the short term, especially when the deficit can be made up relatively quickly through a normal well-balanced diet. But the lack of water in your system is a different matter – especially when repeated studies have shown that it only takes a relatively small degree of dehydration to impair your capacity to perform: as little as 2 per cent of your body weight. The effects? Nausea, dizziness, thirst and, in extreme cases, heat exhaustion, even coma. Dramatic stuff – and

if you forget everything else in this entire chapter, remember one thing: thirst is an unreliable indicator of your state of hydration, so even if you don't 'feel' thirsty or dehydrated during your workout, take a few sips of fluid anyway.

In short, make sure that you drink at least 2.5–3 pints of fluid a day overall and, when getting changed for your step routine about 15–20 minutes before your warm-up, top up your system with a glass. Then take regular sips – little and often – throughout your workout. (One of those cyclist's waterbottles is ideal – especially as it won't spill when you kick it over.) Cool drinks empty more readily from your stomach than warm, so the fluid enters your bloodstream more quickly – not to mention cooling your body down in the process – and large quantities leave your stomach quicker than small – although you should avoid having too much liquid sloshing around inside you when you begin!

Start your rehydration in earnest immediately you stop exercising and don't feel obliged to open a can of 'high-energy' sports drink, since simple water is more than adequate. Most commercial electrolyte drinks contain small quantities of sodium, potassium, chloride and magnesium, as well as the simple sugars, glucose or sucrose, and this dilute solution can help to speed up the whole process of water absorption into your system. Too high a sugar concentration can slow down the process of fluid absorption, though, and also lead to stomach cramps, even nausea, so be careful.

Time to Eat

If you're looking for a good level of energy throughout the day, it stands to reason that you should fuel your body regularly, starting at breakfast. Yes, it's more than tempting to skip this first meal – you haven't got time, you're not hungry, it's an easy meal to cut if you're trying to lose weight, if you start eating that early, you're hungry for the rest of the day . . . But for every excuse for not breaking your fast, there is a better reason why you should.

Lack of time is a poor excuse. How long does it take to drink a glass of juice and have a quick bowl of cereal? And if you do accidentally oversleep, there's no law against eating an apple on the bus and having a tasty bread roll when you get to work. Similarly, who said that breakfast has to be boring old toast and marmalade? Personally, there's nothing I like better than the cold remains of last night's vegetable stew – although even I draw the line at cold curry, not because I can't stomach it but because it's not the most sociable way to enter the office of a morning. Remember, a good nutritious start to the day will keep your energy levels up, and breakfast offers the ideal opportunity to get to work on carbing up for the day ahead.

When it comes to lunchtime, enjoy yourself and again make the most of this opportunity to stock up on carbohydrates. What about a baked potato with cottage cheese or baked beans? After all, both fillings are moist enough to allow you to avoid that dollop of butter completely. Or a good chunky sandwich made from wholemeal bread with a low-fat filling and lashings of salad? If you simply can't exist without some salad dressing, use this to make the bread less dry and simply cut out the margarine. And when it comes to suppertime, think about the carbohydrates first – whether you fancy rice or maybe pasta today – and then add your vegetables or salad before thinking about which fish or meat you'd prefer, or which combination of pulses and nuts you've got most of in the larder. Add heaps of fruit whenever you feel peckish – no point getting too hungry or the quick sugary fix will become all the more tempting – and don't be afraid to have a late-afternoon snack since it's better

to nibble at this point than overeat later on. Sweets and confectionery can then be kept as treats – rather than meal substitutes – and a way of topping up your carbohydrate intake if the pasta and potatoes become too bulky.

The Wasted Workout

That's all very well if you can choose exactly when you exercise. But a lot of people, myself included, work out when they get home at night and then there's the problem of whether you eat something before you start – and risk your supper ending up on your bench in front of you – or hang on until afterwards – and enter the class feeling feeble and half-hearted. A little something extra may be the answer, as much to boost your enthusiasm as anything else.

However, as we've already seen, there is a possibility that eating something sugary before you start could have the opposite effect from what you expected, especially if you haven't been eating plenty of carbohydrates at your other mealtimes. You'll get your initial rush of energy all right as your blood sugar levels surge, but, by the time your workout is really underway, the insulin secreted from your pancreas may well have started to regulate this imbalance by transporting the excess away – an effect enhanced by the very process of exercise itself. Far from feeling bouncy and full of life, you're struggling to keep up, cheating on the movements so that your efforts are wasted, and generally feeling tired, disillusioned and ready to give up. Taken to the extreme, you might even feel dizzy and light-headed.

Watch the Clock

It all boils down to timing. If you need something to boost your energy, avoid anything sugary about three-quarters to half an hour from your starting time – including things like cola and even concentrated fruit juice. The fluid you do need, the sugars you don't. Stoking up either side of this time is fine, though, so what about a cereal bar or banana an hour and a half or so beforehand? Or perhaps you might like to try a little something about five minutes before your warm-up because this doesn't give your pancreas time to secrete its insulin, with the resulting effect. A handful of dried fruit is a snack full of energy which won't weigh heavily on your stomach.

Then, straight after your workout, start refuelling again. It takes on average about two days to restore the fuel to your muscles after exercise, longer in some cases if you've been training particularly hard or if you don't eat enough carbohydrates. However, the glycogen-forming enzymes are at their most active during the first two hours after exercise, so make the most of them and stockpile a good dose in readiness for your next routine.

Food as Fuel

The food we eat has a direct influence on our energy levels and how well we perform. And exercise has a direct influence on the rate at which we burn up our food, not just in the short term, the calorie cost of a given activity, but in the longer term too. For benchwork will help raise your so-called 'basal metabolic rate' – the rate at which your body burns energy when at rest. In other words, step for a few weeks, and your body will not only burn away all that energy during the workouts themselves, but it'll also start burning away more energy when you're not exercising. And you'll still have the luxury of knowing that that loaded plateful of pasta afterwards is both a nutritious, satisfying meal and one which will help make your next workout all the more productive. Which carrot-and-fresh-air diet can do that for you?

So forget about calorie-counting and throw away those scales. After all, that inanimate object in the corner of your bathroom can't differentiate between fat and muscle, or a body which looks lean and well-toned and one which is flabby and out of condition. And whatever you do, do it gradually. A little exercise is better than no exercise – and a few adjustments to your diet are better than none.

chapter twelve

The Next Step

A Few More Thoughts for the Shower

THE SIMPLEST IDEAS are always the best — often the most accessible to the widest number of people, the most effective and the most adaptable. Benchwork is all of these, and *The Ultimate Step* is but an appetizer to what step training is all about. The choreography is kept to the very basics, and there are no exercises involving any of the step bands or straps which can be incorporated in many different ways to focus more on the strength-training side to the workout. Then, of course, there are all the different step programmes in which benchwork has been tailored for the specific training needs of different sports: tennis, skiing and the martial arts, for instance, not to mention aqua-stepping — yes, it appears you can step train underwater! And there's no telling what the next few years will bring.

There's nothing magical about benchwork, though. It's a low-impact form of exercise, with high-impact results. But then again, it's amazing what can be done with a low bench, good music and a desire to take *The Ultimate Step*.

appendix 1

Step to Your Heart's Content

Calculating Your Target Heart Rate

BEFORE STARTING ANY fitness programme it is important to calculate your so-called target heart rate – THR – to ensure that you are working hard enough to benefit from the effects of cardiovascular training, but never so hard that your heart beats at a dangerously high level. For normal healthy individuals, your THR ranges between 65 to 85 per cent of your maximum heart rate, although this upper limit may be a little high for you. Take medical advice if you are in any doubt.

An approximate calculation is simple enough, though, and to begin with you should find your maximum heart rate (MHR):

MHR = 220 − (your age)

So, if you are 30, your MHR will be approximately 190 beats per minute:

MHR = 220 − 30
MHR = 190

Once you have worked this out, multiply that number by 0.65 to find out the lower end of your THR (i.e. 65 per cent):

Lower limit of THR = MHR × 0.65

so for our 30-year-old that will be 123.5 – say 124 – beats per minute (bpm):

190 × 0.65 = 123.5

Then multiply your MHR by 0.85 to establish the upper limit of your THR (i.e. 85 per cent):

Upper limit of THR = MHR × 0.85

so the pulse of our 30-year-old should not exceed 161.5−161 bpm for the sake of argument:

190 × 0.85 = 161.5

Thus, the target heart rate of our 30-year-old is between about 124 and 161 bpm.

The problem is, of course, finding your pulse in the first place. The standard way is to place your index and middle fingers gently on the inside of your wrist, on the artery in line with your thumb. Alternatively, place them gently under your chin just below your back teeth on one side – 'gently' being the operative word here as too much pressure could slow the pulse down. Then, to calculate the number of beats per minute, count how many there are over a ten-second period (you are less likely to lose track!) and multiply that number by six (10 seconds × 6 = 60 seconds or 1 minute).

Realistically, of course, you probably won't have a pen and paper with you, or, indeed, a calculator. So, for ease of reference, the table below provides the average THR in five-year stages for everyone from the age of 20 to 50, including the THR in a ten-second count. All you need to do is remember the upper and lower limit for these ten seconds and compare it to your own ten-second count when you are exercising.

Calculating your THR

Age	MHR	Training Zone* 65%–85%	Training Zone in 10 secs* 65%–85%
20	200	130–170	22–28
25	195	127–166	21–28
30	190	124–161	20–27
35	185	120–157	20–26
40	180	117–153	19–25
45	175	114–149	19–25
50	170	110–145	18–24

*Note: These figures are only an approximate guide for healthy individuals. If you want to find out your exact THR you must consult your doctor. For people whose ages fall between the five-year segments, use the figures for the next age group up (i.e. if you are 27, take the THR of an average 30-year-old).

Take your pulse for the first time once you think that you have warmed up – if you have, it should have reached the lower end of your THR – then take it again after about 10 minutes of stepping, to check that you're not overdoing things but aren't being lazy. Whatever you do, however, do not just stop dead when you take your pulse. Keep marching on the spot so that you don't cool down too much or allow the blood to pool in your legs and so make you feel dizzy. Then, when you have finished your workout, check your pulse regularly, to check your recovery rate. If it takes longer than normal to slow down, it means that you have probably been overdoing things and should ease back a bit next time.

Remember, the THR of 65–85 per cent is only a rough guideline and your body is absolutely correct if it tells you to keep to the lower end of the scale and not overdo things. The aim is to build up your level of fitness gradually over the next few months – and any exercise is better than none.

The Perceived Rate of Exertion

There are problems with having to take your pulse all the time, though – not least of which being the fact that it disrupts your workout. Not only is it sometimes difficult to locate your pulse quickly and accurately, but it's all too easy to miscount the number of beats and so have to start again – by which time your heart rate will be slower and the reading inaccurate. Nevertheless, it is worth persevering with for a while because after a few weeks you will be able to tell instinctively whether you are working within acceptable limits or not, just by listening to your body.

This is precisely the time when it would be a good idea to combine this method of intensity measurement with a second, less complicated approach known as Perceived Rate of Exertion – or PRE for short. As its name suggests, this is a subjective way of assessing heart rate and oxygen intake, originally using a scale of 6–20 with a verbal description for each: 6, for example, being 'very, very light'; between 11 ('fairly light') and 13 ('somewhat hard') correlating to about 60–65 per cent of the maximum heart rate; and 15 ('hard') representing about 90 per cent. If you reached 19 ('very, very hard') when you were really struggling and your breathing became extremely difficult, it was definitely time to put the brakes on, as you were nearly at your maximum heart rate (ACSM, *Guidelines*). This scale was later modified for ease of use, though, so that it now ranges from 1–10 and is a simple but effective way to gauge your training intensity. Aim at working somewhere between a 'moderate' demand on your body and a 'heavy' demand, and double-check this every so often by taking your pulse.

appendix 2

The Routines in Brief

The First-timer's Routine (Chapter Six)

Repeat each step 16 times on each side. If no indication is given about arm movements, pump them vigorously at your sides.

1. Step, leading right
   TAP DOWN
   Step leading left
   TAP DOWN

2. Step leading right – with half-speed bicep curls
   TAP DOWN
   Step leading left – with full-speed bicep curls
   TAP DOWN

3. Step leading right – with half-speed up-right rows
   TAP DOWN
   Step leading left – with full-speed upright rows
   TAP DOWN

4. V-step leading right – hands on hips
   TAP DOWN
   V-step leading left – with flyes
   TAP DOWN

5. Wide step leading right
   TAP DOWN
   Wide step leading left
   TAP DOWN

6. V-step leading right

7. TAP DOWN into alternate tap down – with half-speed alternate tricep kick-back

8. Alternate tap down in the centre – with full-speed tricep kick-back

9. Step leading right – with bicep curl
   TAP DOWN
   Step leading left – with tricep kick-back
   TAP DOWN

10. Step leading right
    TAP DOWN
    Step leading left

11. TAP UP right into alternate tap up

12. Add chest press

13. Alternate knee lift – with bicep curl

14. Alternate leg curl – with tricep kick-back

15. Alternate side leg – with lat raises or flyes

16. Alternate tap up

17. Alternate knee lifts – with pec deck

18. Alternate tap up

19. Step leading right – with chest press
    KNEE LIFT

20. Step leading left
    TAP DOWN
    Step leading right
    TAP DOWN
    Step leading left

March behind bench

Turning Up the Heat – The Face-on Routine (Chapter Seven)

1. Sixteen steps leading right – with bicep curl
   TAP DOWN
   Sixteen steps leading left – with tricep kick-back

2. Eight alternate tap ups leading right
   Sixteen alternate knee lifts – with chest press and thigh touch

3. Eight travelling knee lifts – with shoulder press

4. Four sets of three travelling knee lifts – with lateral pull-down

5. Four sets of three adductor touches – touch foot
   Four sets of three leg curls – with tricep kick-back
   Four sets of three side legs – with lat raises
   Four sets of three buttock bashers

6. Eight travelling tap ups

7. Eight shuffles – with chest press/shoulder press

8. Four travelling knee lifts
   Eight alternate tap ups facing the front

9. Eight steps leading right
   TAP DOWN
   Eight steps leading left
   TAP DOWN

10. Eight V-steps leading right – with arms following legs
    TAP DOWN
    Eight V-steps leading left – with arms following legs
    TAP DOWN

11. Sixteen alternate V-steps – with double-time arms

12. Sixteen turn steps – with chest press

13. Eight turn steps with a lunge – with press-and-punch arms

14. Four reps of three lunges – with press-and-punch arms

15. Seven turn steps

Squat behind bench facing right

Turning Up the Heat – The Side-on Routine

Squat behind bench facing right

1. Sixteen traverses

2. Sixteen traverses with a knee lift – climb the rope!

3. Four traverses with reps of five knee lifts – with pec deck

4. Eight traverses with single knee lifts and straddle – with chest press

5. Eight traverses with single knee lifts and squats – with chest and shoulder presses
or
Eight traverses with single knee lifts and straddle – with chest and shoulder presses

6. Four traverses with single knee lifts and straddle
Eight straddles leading left – climb the rope!
TAP UP
Eight straddles leading right – climb the rope!

7. Eight alternate lunges – with single arm chest press

8. Eight sets of four lunges – with single arm shoulder press

9. Eight single lunges – with single arm chest press

10. Eight straddles leading left – with lat raises
TAP UP
Eight straddles leading right – with lat raises

11. TAP UP
Sixteen alternate straddle steps – with upright rows

12. Eight alternate squats – with shoulder press
or
Eight straddle steps with a knee lift – with bicep curl

13. Sixteen alternate straddle steps

14. Single lunges with alternate straddles – repeated eight times

15. Eight traverses leading right – with tricep kick-back

Squat behind bench facing right

Turning Up the Heat – The End-on Routine

Squat behind bench facing right

1. Eight traverses leading left – with chest press

2. Eight straddles leading left – climb the rope!
TAP UP
Eight straddles leading right – climb the rope!
(Move to back of bench)
TAP UP

3. Eight T-steps leading left – with pec deck
TAP DOWN
Eight T-steps leading right – with pec deck
TAP DOWN

4. Sixteen alternate T-steps – with flyes

5. Sixteen alternate T-steps with side leg and buttock basher – with lat raises

6. Sixteen alternate T-steps – alternating two pec decks and two flyes

7. Eight straddle steps leading right – with bicep curls
TAP UP
Eight straddle steps leading left – with tricep kick-back
TAP UP

8. Sixteen alternate lunges – with single arm chest press

9. STEP OFF RIGHT
Eight traverses leading left

10. Eight traverses with a knee lift — with chest press

11. Eight traverses with a knee lift and straddle/squat — with shoulder press

12. Eight traverses with knee lift
Eight traverses

13. STEP OFF RIGHT AND FACE FRONT
Eight steps leading left
TAP DOWN
Eight steps leading right
TAP DOWN

14. Sixteen alternate V-steps — with arms following legs

15. Sixteen alternate tap downs in centre

Squat behind bench

The Crunching Routine (Chapter Eight)

1. Eight steps leading right
TAP DOWN
Eight steps leading left

2. TAP UP
Four alternate knee lifts leading into travelling knee lifts

3. Four alternate knee lifts — with bent-arm back squeeze
Four alternate knee lifts — with skier
Alternate the above four more times

4. Four alternate tap ups — with marionette back push
Four alternate tap ups — with marionette
Alternate the above four more times

5. Eight alternate tap ups — shaking out arms

6. Four alternate tap ups — with pec deck
Four alternate tap ups — with chest squeeze
Alternate the above four times more

7. Four alternate tap ups — with straight-arm pulse
Four alternate tap ups — with straight-arm forward push
Alternate the above four times more

8. STEP OFF BENCH AND SQUAT WITH FEET APART. SHAKE ARMS.

9. Four sets of four slow half-step squats on alternate sides — with straight-arm back pulse

10. Four slow full step squats leading right
TAP DOWN
Four slow full step squats leading left
TAP DOWN

11. Eight alternate V-steps

12. Eight tap up-tap downs leading right
Eight tap up-tap downs leading left

13. Eight knee lift-lunges leading right
Eight knee lift-lunges leading left

14. Step leading right to right-hand end of bench
TAP DOWN
The crusher — with eight singles
four reps of three
two reps of five
two reps of three
four singles

15. Step leading left to left-hand end of bench
TAP DOWN
The crusher — as above

16. Sixteen steps leading right
TAP DOWN
Sixteen steps leading left

Squat behind bench

glossary

The first full description of each term or exercise is given in brackets.

Abdominals (abs) – the stomach muscles

Adductors – the muscles down the inner thigh

Adductor Touch – using your hand to touch your foot while easing a knee lift across your body (see p 50)

Alternating – any step in which the leading leg changes every time

Biceps – the muscle at the front of the upper arm

Climb the Rope – a scissors arm movement (see pp 46–7)

Crunch – an abdominal exercise in which you lie on the floor with your feet raised and knees bent, and squeeze your stomach muscles to lift your shoulders a couple of inches off the ground (see p 93)

Curl – a movement which involves bending a joint in order to work a given muscle or muscle group: hence, *bicep curl* (see p 37), working the upper arm, and *leg curl* (see pp 34–5), working the back of the thigh. Also an abdominal exercise in which you lie on the floor with your knees bent and feet flat, and contract your stomach muscles to lift your shoulders a couple of inches off the floor (see pp 91–2).

Flye – a hugging movement to exercise the chest (see pp 90–91)

Gluteals – the muscles in the buttocks

Hamstring – the muscles at the back of the thigh

Lateral (lat) raises – a sideways movement with the arms to work the upper back and shoulders (see p 39)

Leading leg – the leg which steps up on to the bench first

Lunge – a strong movement in which alternate legs are extended behind you and back again (see pp 54–6)

Pec deck – a hugging movement similar to the flye which works the chest (see p 41)
Pectorals (pecs) – the main chest muscles
Press – a pushing action with the arms: hence, *chest press* (see p 40), pushing both arms out to the front at chest height, and *shoulder press* (see pp 49–50), pushing both arms above the head
Pulse – a small controlled movement which takes just one beat (see p 92)

Quadriceps (quads) – the muscles down the front of the thigh

Repeaters (reps) – an action repeated three or five times in succession on the same side (see p 50)

Set – a group of movements
Shuffle – a travelling step which uses both the length and the end of the bench (see pp 48–9)
Straddle – a step starting on top of the bench in which you step down on either side then up again (see pp 56–9)
Squat – a movement in which both knees are bent and straightened again, either with the feet together (as at the start of the routines) or apart. There is also the *straddle/squat* (see

p 57), where the bench is between the legs, or the *slow squat* (see pp 69–71), where one foot is on the bench, one on the floor.

Tap down – the movement to change the leading leg in which the trailing foot taps the floor and steps up again straight away (see p 33)
Tap up – the movement to change the leading leg in which the trailing foot taps the top of the bench and steps off again straight away (see p 33)
Trailing leg – the leg which reaches the bench after the first leg
Traverse – a movement which crosses the bench from the side (see pp 54–5)
Tricep kick-back – a downward-pressing movement which works the triceps (see pp 38–9)
Triceps – the muscles at the back of the upper arm

Upright rows – an upward-pulling movement in which the hands are together and elbows high (see pp 39–40)

V-step – a movement in which the feet are placed at either end on the bench when you step up, and brought back together again as you step off (see p 36)

Wide step – a development of the V-step in which the feet remain apart as you step off (see p 36)